PUBLIC HEALTH: PRACTICES, METHODS AND POLICIES

MEASLES

EPIDEMIOLOGY AND CONTROL OF MEASLES IN THE GWERU URBAN DISTRICT IN ZIMBABWE

PUBLIC HEALTH: PRACTICES, METHODS AND POLICIES

Series Editor: Joav Merrick, Medical Director, Health Services, Division for Intellectual and Developmental Disabilities, Ministry of Social Affairs and Social Services, Jerusalem, Israel

Environment and Public Health: Environmental Health, Law and International Perspectives
I. Leslie Rubin and Joav Merrick (Editors)
2014. ISBN: 978-1-63463-167-9 (Hardcover)

Tomorrow's Leaders: Service Leadership and Holistic Development in Chinese University Students
Daniel T.L. Shek, Andrew M.H. Siu and Joav Merrick (Editors)
2015. ISBN: 978-1-63321-880-2 (Hardcover)

Arbovirus: Public Health Experience from Zambia
Seter Siziya, Ph.D., Mazyanga L. Mazaba, Joav Merrick, M.D. (Editors)
2015. ISBN: 978-1-63463-601-8 (Hardcover)

Health Issues in Diverse Cultures
Cecilia Obeng, Samuel Gyasi Obeng and Joav Merrick (Editors)
2015. ISBN: 978-1-63463-613-1 (Hardcover)

Public Health, Social Work and Health Inequalities
Bruce D. Friedman, Ph.D. and Joav Merrick, M.D. (Editors)
2015. ISBN: 978-1-63482-838-3 (Hardcover)

Environmental Health Disparities: Costs and Benefits of Breaking the Cycle
I. Leslie Rubin, M.D., and Joav Merrick, M.D. (Editors)
2016. ISBN: 978-1-63484-211-2 (Hardcover)

Smoking and Adolescence: International Public Health Experiences
Mazyanga L. Mazaba, Seter Siziya, Ph.D., Joav Merrick, M.D. (Editors)
2016. ISBN: 978-1-63484-311-9 (Hardcover)

Public Health: Some International Aspects
Joav Merrick, M.D. (Editor)
2016. ISBN: 978-1-63484-612-7 (Hardcover)

Medical History: Some Perspectives
Donald E. Greydanus, and Joav Merrick (Editors)
2016. ISBN: 978-1-63484-747-6 (Hardcover)

Public Health: International Aspects on Environment and Health
I. Leslie Rubin, M.D., and Joav Merrick, M.D.(Editors)
2016. ISBN: 978-1-63484-834-3 (Hardcover)

Education in Hong Kong: Service Leadership for University Students
Daniel TL Shek, Cecilia Ma, Li Lin, and Joav Merrick
2016. ISBN: 978-1-63484-928-9 (Hardcover)

Higher Education in Hong Kong: Nurturing Students to be Caring Service Leaders
Daniel TL Shek, Andrew MH Siu, Hildie Leung, and Joav Merrick (Editors)
2016. ISBN: 978-1-63484-980-7 (Hardcover)

Measles: Epidemiology and Control of Measles in the Gweru Urban District in Zimbabwe
Tawanda Marufu, Seter Siziya, Mazyanga L. Mazaba and Joav Merrick (Editors)
2016. ISBN: 978-1-63485-559-4 (Softcover)

PUBLIC HEALTH: PRACTICES, METHODS AND POLICIES

MEASLES

EPIDEMIOLOGY AND CONTROL OF MEASLES IN THE GWERU URBAN DISTRICT IN ZIMBABWE

TAWANDA MARUFU
SETER SIZIYA
MAZYANGA L MAZABA
AND
JOAV MERRICK
EDITORS

New York

Library of Congress Cataloging-in-Publication Data

Library of Congress Control Number: 2016942398
ISBN: 978-1-63485-559-4

Published by Nova Science Publishers, Inc. † New York

CONTENTS

Introduction 1

Chapter 1 Introduction to the epidemiology and control of measles in Gweru City Urban District in Zimbabwe 3
Tawanda Marufu, Seter Siziya, Mazyanga L. Mazaba and Joav Merrick

Section one: Epidemiology of measles 1960-1989 11

Chapter 2 Impact of vaccination on measles transmission patterns 13
Tawanda Marufu, Seter Siziya and Willard Tinago

Chapter 3 Changes in rates of measles transmission and force of infection 27
Tawanda Marufu, Willard Tinago and Seter Siziya

Chapter 4 Challenges posed by changes in measles transmission patterns 35
Tawanda Marufu, Seter Siziya, Mufuta Tshimanga, Elizabeth Xaba, Chris Ruwodo, Zenzo Silape, Tsitsi Baye and Melisa Hhlazo

Chapter 5 Questioning the level of efficacy of the measles vaccine in use in Zimbabwe **45**
Tawanda Marufu, Seter Siziya, Boniface Manyame, Elizabeth Xaba, Zenzo Silape, Perpetua Zimbizi, Chris Ruwodo, Elizabeth Mason, Reginald B Matchaba-Hove and Oliver Mudyarabikwa

Section two: Use of multiple dose measles vaccination strategies in the control of measles **53**

Chapter 6 Impact of multiple dose measles vaccination on measles transmission patterns **55**
Tawanda Marufu and Seter Siziya

Chapter 7 Comparison of protection afforded by single measles vaccination and late revaccination schedules **63**
Tawanda Marufu, Seter Siziya, Mufuta Tshimanga, Shiva Murugasampillay and Elizabeth Mason

Chapter 8 Comparison of impact of single dose and multiple dose measles vaccination strategies on measles transmission patterns **71**
Tawanda Marufu, Seter Siziya and Willard Tinago

Section three: Complicated measles and mortality **81**

Chapter 9 Factors associated with secular trends in mortality attributed to measles **83**
Tawanda Marufu, Seter Siziya and Kaka Mudambo

Chapter 10 Factors associated with measles complications **95**
Tawanda Marufu, Seter Siziya, Mufuta Tshimanga, Shiva Murugasampillay, Elizabeth Mason and Boniface Manyame

Chapter 11 Secular changes in rates of respiratory complications and diarrhoea among measles cases **105**
Tawanda Marufu and Seter Siziya

Chapter 12 Impact of malnutrition and measles mortality on children under five years of age **113**
Tawanda Marufu, Seter Siziya and Willard Tinago

Section four: Acknowledgments 123

Chapter 13 About the editors 125

Chapter 14 About the College of Health Sciences at the University of Zimbabwe 129

Chapter 15 About the School of Medicine, Copperbelt University in Ndola, Zambia 133

Chapter 16 About the National Institute of Child Health and Human Development in Israel 137

Chapter 17 About the book series "Public health: Practices, methods and policies" 141

Section five: Index 143

Index 145

INTRODUCTION

In: Measles
Editors: T. Marufu, S. Siziya et al.
ISBN: 978-1-63485-559-4

Chapter 1

INTRODUCTION TO THE EPIDEMIOLOGY AND CONTROL OF MEASLES IN GWERU CITY URBAN DISTRICT IN ZIMBABWE

Tawanda Marufu*[1], *MB ChB, MSc,
Seter Siziya*[2], *BA(Ed), MSc, PhD,
Mazyanga L. Mazaba*[3], *BSc, MSc
and Joav Merrick*[4-8], *MD, MMedSci, DMSc

[1]Department of Community Medicine, University of Zimbabwe College of Health Sciences in Harare, Zimbabwe
[2]Department of Clinical Sciences, Copperbelt University, Ndola, Zambia
[3]Expanded Program on Immunisation (EPI), World Health Organization, Lusaka, Zambia
[4]National Institute of Child Health and Human Development, Jerusalem, Israel
[5]Office of the Medical Director, Health Services, Division for Intellectual and Developmental Disabilities, Ministry of Social Affairs and Social Services, Jerusalem, Israel
[6]Division of Pediatrics, Hadassah Hebrew University Medical Center, Mt Scopus Campus, Jerusalem, Israel
[7]Kentucky Children's Hospital, University of Kentucky College of Medicine, Lexington, Kentucky, United States of America
[8]Center for Healthy Development, School of Public Health, Georgia State University, Atlanta, United States of America

INTRODUCTION

Mortality attributed to measles declined in 1967-1989 in Gweru city (1, 2). Factors that were associated with this decline included good management of complicated measles cases (1, 2) and decline in malnutrition among children aged <5 years (2). These findings contradict those of other studies that have attributed major declines in measles mortality in Africa to supplementary measles immunization activities (SIAs) that were applied in 1996 and after (3, 4). In Zimbabwe, as was found in Gweru, data on secular trends in measles mortality dating way back before SIAs seem to indicate that decline in measles mortality that was observed post application of SIAs would have been a continuation of a trend that had commenced a lot earlier (5).

In 1960-1989 decline in measles and malnutrition mortality among underfives in Gweru city accounted for 70.5% variation in the decline of all-cause underfives mortality in the same period (6). This is very much unlike other developing countries where in 2000-03 it was estimated that neonatal disorders, pneumonia and diarrhoea accounted for 73% of all underfives mortality while malaria, measles, HIV/AIDS, injuries and other causes accounted for the remaining 27% (7). The explanation for differences in the findings from Gweru and estimates from other developing countries were thought to arise from the fact that major causes of underfives mortality are period specific (as in time or era) (8) and area specific (as in geographical distribution) (7, 9).

CHANGES IN MEASLES TRANSMISSION PATTERNS

Measles vaccination was commenced in Gweru in 1971. In 1971-1989 a single dose of live hyper-attenuated Schwartz strain vaccine (0.5mls or 1000 $TCID_{50}$) was administered to children at 9 months of age at the city's six primary care health facilities. At vaccine coverage rates of >90% in 1986-89 measles incidence rates significantly declined (10). This was very much like experiences elsewhere where sustained high vaccine coverage rates led to decline in measles transmission (11-13).

Among reported measles cases, vaccinated cases (vaccine failures) significantly increased as vaccine coverage rates increased such that in 1980-1989 more than 51% of all reported measles cases were vaccine failures. (10, 14) Occurrence of vaccine failures is blamed on a vaccine of less that 100%

efficacy (15-18). Accumulation of vaccine failures in developing countries with moderate to high measles vaccine coverage rates has led to epidemics after a decline in measles transmission (18, 19). Public health and policy issues that would arise from this were that, although measles transmission was declining in Gweru city on account of high vaccine coverage rates (10, 14), it would not be possible to sustain the declining transmission and also it would not be possible to either eliminate (20-22) or eradicate measles in this setting (23-25).

Measles vaccine efficacy studies carried out in Gweru in 1987-89 found an efficacy of 77% for the vaccine that is applied to children at 9 months of age (17). This meant that for every 100 children that are vaccinated some 80% or less would get immunized leaving 20% or so unprotected. Low level of vaccine efficacy found in Gweru was similar to that found in studies in other developing countries or areas (26-28). This level of efficacy was thought to be due to effects of transplacentally acquired maternal antibodies that would not have decayed at time the vaccine is applied to children at 9 months of age (17, 28).

As vaccine coverage rates increased in Gweru the disease shifted from younger age groups of <59 months to older children of aged > 60 months (10, 14). The shift of the disease to these older children was associated with significant increased susceptibility (increased risk) of contracting measles by this age group compared to younger age groups of <59 months (14, 29, 30) This high susceptibility to infection was found to be due to accumulation of vaccine failures in this age group. (14, 29) Shift of disease from younger to older age groups which is associated with accumulation of vaccine failures in the older age groups (as was found in Gweru) has occurred in some developing countries with high vaccine coverage rates of measles vaccine that is applied at 9 months of age (31-34). Measles epidemics that have occurred in some developing countries and areas in communities and schools have mostly involved children that are >60 months of age most of whom had had vaccination (19, 32, 35). What this meant is that measles was now occurring at ages for which no immunization policy existed because the only policy that was operational was that of applying vaccine at 9 months age and yet there was now an obvious need to vaccinate these older age groups to avert epidemics in the future.

The Multiple -Dose Measles Vaccination Project in Gweru, 1990-1996

Two basic principles underpinned the multiple-dose vaccination project in Gweru: (a) Application of another dose of measles vaccine (after the dose that is applied at 9 months of age) at a point in time when it is assumed that all maternal antibodies will have decayed, would improve vaccine efficacy thereby reducing occurrence of vaccine failures, and (b) By the late 1980s vaccine coverage rates where >90% but on account of the low efficacy for the vaccine applied at 9 months of age most measles transmission was sustained by vaccine failures. To undo vaccine failures that had accumulated over the years there was a need to mount a mass vaccination campaign in the population within the age range where most measles transmission occurred i.e., children aged 10-119 months. Because we were going to vaccinate these children irrespective of disease history or vaccination status, obviously children that had not had vaccination were also going to be netted in this effort and this therefore enabled us to further reduce the pool of susceptibles.

The measles multiple dose project in Gweru city was run over a period of seven years, 1990-1996. In early 1990 over a two-week period a mass vaccination campaign was carried out among children aged 10-119 months. Vaccine was applied to these children irrespective of disease history or vaccination status. For the rest of the project period (after this campaign) children that had vaccination at 9 months of age were provided another single dose (revaccination) at any point in time between ages of 12 and 23 moths (33, 34). The project was run as a quasi-experimental community intervention that had both an ‘internal’ and an ‘external’ comparisons. The ‘internal’ comparison compared measles transmission patterns in Gweru in 1983-1989 (seven years prior to the intervention) and 1990-1996 (the intervention period). Measles transmission patterns in Gweru city were compared with those of Bulawayo city, the ‘external’ comparison, in 1983-89 and in 1990-1996. Bulawayo was specifically selected to be the external comparison because (a) age structure of populations in Gweru and Bulawayo were similar and so were the living conditions, (b) structures for measles surveillance and monitoring of measles vaccinations in Bulawayo were similar to those of Gweru, and (c) up till 1990 Bulawayo, like Gweru, had maintained high measles vaccine coverage rates (>85%) for the vaccine applied at 9 months of age and had the capacity to sustain these rates during the project period, 1990-1996. In Gweru, over and above comparisons of impact of single dose and multiple dose vaccination strategies between the 'external' and 'internal' comparisons, over a five year period 1990-1994 studies were carried out to determine and compare vaccine efficacies for the single dose vaccination and multiple dose vaccination schedules (36).

In the project period (1990-1994) vaccine efficacy found for the vaccine applied at nine months of age was 77.2% (36) which was not any different from the 77% found in studies carried out in Gweru 1987-89 (17). Efficacy of vaccine applied at ages 12-23 months was found to be 96.6% (36) and it was concluded that late revaccination afforded vaccinees better protection than single vaccination applied at 9 months of age.

In Gweru in 1990-1996 measles transmission was significant lower than in 1993-1989 and this decline was associated with a major reduction in vaccine failures particularly among older age groups of 60-119 months (33). In Bulawayo, despite high measles vaccine coverage rates of >90%, there were measles epidemics in1992, 1993, 1994 and 1996 even when in the earlier period (1983-1989) measles incidence rates had been declining precipitously. The epidemics of measles experienced in 1990-96 were associated with high transmission of measles in children aged >60 months most of whom were vaccine failures (34).

The city of Gweru multiple dose measles vaccination project was presented at the Fourth International Seminar on Immunization in Africa in Yamoussoukro, Ivory Coast, in 1994 when the project had been operational for five years with two more years to go (37). It was the only project of its nature (on measles multiple dose vaccination) being run in Africa at the time and at this conference this was the first time the international public health community got to know about the project. The principles behind the project and results of the project up till that time were indicated in the presentation. WHO representatives at the meeting could not contest the scientific basis of the project (including the results) but insisted that they would still go by the policy of application of vaccine at 9 months of age only despite overwhelming evidence of a need for policy change (38). However, since 2001 WHO and UNICEF have embraced the principle of multiple dose measles vaccination (39, 40) and this is particularly so in response to the worldwide movement towards measles elimination (20-22) and eradication (23-25). High measles vaccine coverage with multiple dose vaccination (in the form of routine two-dose vaccination applied to children at 9 months and after 12 months of age, and occasional supplementary immunization activities applied nationally or in at risk areas/population groups) coupled with case based measles surveillance and a well-articulated measles epidemic control effort would be the most basic public health/epidemiological armourmentarium required for elimination and eradication of measles in developing countries.

REFERENCES

[1] Marufu T, Siziya S, Murugasampillay S, Mason E, Manyame B, Tshimanga M. Measles complication: the importance of their management in reducing mortality attributed to measles. Cent Afr J Med 1997;43:162-5.

[2] Marufu T, Siziya S, Mudambo KS. Factors associated with secular trends in mortality attributed to measles in Gweru, Zimbabwe, in 1967-1989. J Trop Pediatr 2008;54:114-9.

[3] Biellik R, Madema S, Taole A, Kutsulukuta A, Allies E, Eggers R, et al. First 5 years of measles elimination in southern Africa: 1996-2000. Lancet 2002;359:1564-8.

[4] Otten M, Kezaala R, Fall A, Masresha B, Martin R, Cairns L, et al. Public-health impact of accelerated measles control in the WHO African Region 2000-03. Lancet 2005;366:832-9.

[5] Marufu T, Siziya S, Tinago W. Secular trends in mortality attributed to measles in Zimbabwe. Unpublished manuscript.

[6] Marufu T, Siziya S, Tinago W. Impact of malnutrition and measles mortality on underfives all-cause mortality in Gweru City, Zimbabwe, in 1960-89. Eur J Prev Med 2015;3:209-12.

[7] Bryce J, Boschi-Pinto C, Shibuya K, Black RE, WHO Child Health Epidemiology Reference Group. WHO estimates of the causes of death in children. Lancet 2005;365:1147-52.

[8] Caulfield LE, de Onis M, Blossner M, Black RE. Undernutrition as an underlying cause of child deaths associated with diarrhea, pneumonia, malaria, and measles. Am J Clin Nutr 2004;80:193-8.

[9] Black RE, Morris SS, Bryce J. Where and why are 10 million children dying every year? Lancet 2003;361:2226-34.

[10] Marufu T, Siziya S, Tinago W. Impact of vaccination on measles transmission patterns in Gweru city, Zimbabwe, 1960-89. Eur J Prev Med 2016;4:65-72.

[11] Centers for Disease Control and Prevention (CDC). Global measles mortality, 2000-2008. MMWR 2009;58:1321-6.

[12] Keeling MJ, Rhani P. Modelling infectious diseases in humans and animals. Princeton, NJ: Princeton University Press, 2008.

[13] Goldhaber-Fiebert JD, Lipsitch M, Mahal A, Zaslavsky AM, Salomon JA. Quantifying child mortality reductions related to measles vaccination. PLoS One 2010;5:e13842.

[14] Marufu T. The changing age ecology of measles and its implications on measles control. Cent Afr J Med 1992; 38:208-14.

[15] Rosenthal SR, Clements CJ. Two-dose measles vaccination schedules. Bull World Health Organ 1993;71:421-8.

[16] Marufu T, Siziya S, Tshimanga M, Xaba E, Ruwodo C, Silape Z, et al. Challenges posed by changes in measles transmission patterns. Cent Afr J Med 1998;44:5-8.

[17] Marufu T, Siziya S, Manyame B, Xaba E, Silape-Marufu Z, Zimbizi P, et al. Questioning the level of efficacy of the measles vaccine in use in Zimbabwe. Cent Afr J Med 1995;41:241-5.
[18] Global Programme for Vaccines and Immunization. Immunization policy. Expanded programme on immunization. Geneva: WHO/EPI/GEN/92.3, 1995.
[19] Coetzee N, Hussey GD, Visser G, Barron P, Keen A. The 1992 measles epidemic in Cape Town-a changing epidemiological pattern. S Afr Med J 1994;84:145-9
[20] de Quadros CA1, Olivé JM, Hersh BS, Strassburg MA, Henderson DA, Brandling-Bennett D, Alleyne GA. Measles elimination in the Americas. Evolving strategies. JAMA 1996;275: 224-9.
[21] Cutts FT, Lessler J, Metcalf CJ. Measles elimination: progress, challenges and implications for rubella control. Expert Rev Vaccines 2013;12:917-32.
[22] Anonymous. Meeting of the Strategic Advisory Group of Experts on Immunization, November 2012 - conclusions and recommendations. Wkly Epidemiol Rec 2013;88:1-16.
[23] Moss WJ, Strebel P. Biological feasibility of measles eradication. J Infect Dis 2011;204(Supp l)1:S47-53.
[24] de Quadros CA, Andrus JK, Danovaro-Holliday MC, Castillo-Solórzano C. Feasibility of global measles eradication after interruption of transmission in the Americas. Expert Rev Vaccines 2008;7:355-62.
[25] Andrus JK, de Quadros CA, Solorzano CC, Periago MR, Henderson DA. Measles and rubella eradication in the Americas. Vaccine 2011;29(Suppl 4):D91-6.
[26] Kambarami RA, Nathoo KJ, Nkrumah FK, Pirie DJ. Measles epidemic in Harare, Zimbabwe, despite high measles immunization coverage rates. Bull World Health Organ 1991;69:213-9.
[27] Mudzamiri WS, Peterson DE, Marufu T, Biellick RJ, L'Herminez M. Measles vaccine efficacy in Masvingo district, Zimbabwe. Cent Afr J Med 1996;42:195-7.
[28] Foster S, McFarland DA. Measles. In: Jamison DT, Mosley HW, eds. The World Bank health sector priorities review. Washington, DC: World Bank, 1991:10-11.
[29] Marufu T, Tinago W, Siziya S. Changes in rates of measles transmission and force of infection in Gweru city, Zimbabwe: A retrospective study. Eur J Prev Med 2016;4:28-31
[30] Marufu T, Murugasampillary S, Siziya S, Manyame B, Silape-Marufu Z, Xaba E, et al. Is the protection afforded measles vaccinees the same in children of all age groups? Cent Afr J Med 1995;41:144-7.
[31] Expanded Programme on Immunization Measles control in the 1990s: Plan of action for global measles control. Geneva: WHO/EPI/GEN/92.3, 1992.
[32] Cutts FT. Measles control in the 1990s: Principles for the next decade. Geneva: WHO/EPI/GEN 90.2, 1990.
[33] Marufu T, Siziya S. Impact of multiple dose measles vaccination on measles transmission patterns in Gweru, Zimbabwe. J Trop Pediatr 2001;47:335-8.
[34] Marufu T, Siziya S, Tinago W. Comparison of single dose and multiple dose measles vaccination strategies on measles transmission patterns. Eur J Prev Med 2015;3:80-4.
[35] Khuri-Bulos NA. Measles in Jordan: a prototype of the problems with measles in developing countries. Pediatr Infect Dis J 1995;14:22-6.

[36] Marufu T, Siziya S, Tshimanga M, Murugasampillay S, Mason E. Comparison of protection afforded by single measles vaccination and late revaccination schedules. East Afr Med J 1997;74:777-9.

[37] Marufu T, Silape Z, Xaba E, Zimbizi P, Shearley A. Measles revaccination project in the city of Gweru 1990-1994: Impact of the Two-dose measles vaccination schedule in the city of Gweru, Zimbabwe, 1990-1992. 4th International Seminar on Immunizations in Africa, Yamoussoukro – Cote D'Ivoire, 13-16 Mar 1994:86-92.

[38] Summary of discussions and principal conclusions (on booster vaccination doses). 4th International Seminar on Immunizations in Africa, Yamoussoukro – Cote D'Ivoire, 13-16 Mar 1994:101-102.

[39] Goodson JL, Masresha BG, Wannemuehler K, Uzicanin A, Cochi S. Changing epidemiology of measles in Africa. J Infect Dis. 2011;204(Suppl 1):S205-14.

[40] World Health Organization and UNICEF. Measles mortality reduction and regional elimination: Strategic plan 2001-2005. URL: http://www.who.int/vaccines-documents/DocsPDF01/www573.pdf.

SECTION ONE: EPIDEMIOLOGY OF MEASLES 1960-1989

In: Measles
Editors: T. Marufu, S. Siziya et al.
ISBN: 978-1-63485-559-4

Chapter 2

IMPACT OF VACCINATION ON MEASLES TRANSMISSION PATTERNS

Tawanda Marufu[1,*], MB ChB, MSc, Seter Siziya[2], BA(Ed), MSc, PhD and Willard Tinago[1], BSc, MSc, PhD

[1]Department of Community Medicine,
University of Zimbabwe College of Health Sciences,
Harare, Zimbabwe
[2]Department of Clinical Sciences,
Copperbelt University School of Medicine,
Ndola, Zambia

A study was carried out in Gweru city urban district (population-158233) in Zimbabwe to determine the impact of measles vaccine applied at 9 months of age on measles transmission patterns. A retrospective observational study that used data from measles vaccination records and measles disease surveillance was conducted. Linear regression analysis and the chi-squared test for linear trend (χ^2) were used to investigate linear relationships at a 5% significance level. Vaccine coverage rates were 0% in pre-vaccination era in 1960-70 and 2-92% in1971-89 (median=65, Q_1=34, Q_3=88) when they significantly linearly increased ($p<0.001$). In 1960-85 measles incidence rates significantly linearly

* Correspondence: Tawanda Marufu, University of Zimbabwe College of Health Sciences, Box A 178, Avondale, Harare, Zimbabwe. E-mail: marufut@yahoo.com.

increased ($p<0.001$) while in 1986-89 at vaccine coverage rates of >90% incidence rates significantly linearly declined ($p<0.001$). Proportion of vaccinated cases among measles notifications significantly linearly increased as vaccine coverage rates increased (Slope: +1.19, 95% CI [0.52, 1.86]). At vaccine coverage rates of >80% (1984-89), proportion of vaccine failures among cases aged 60-119 months was significantly higher than at vaccine coverage rates of <80% (1971-83) ($p=0.011$) while in age group 10-59 months proportions of vaccine failures were not different at vaccine coverage rates of <80% and >80%. In age group 60-119 months incidence rates significantly linearly increased as vaccine coverage rates increased (Slope: +29.88, 95 CI [13.95, 45.82]). In pre-vaccination era, and at vaccine coverage rates of <80% and >80% some 75% of all reported measles cases occurred by age 36-47 months, 48-59 months and 72-83 months respectively. In conclusion, measles incidence rates declined at vaccine coverage rates of >90%, while measles vaccine failures significantly increased as vaccine coverage rates increased. Increasing measles vaccination coverage led to shift of age at infection from age group <59 months to age group 60-119 months and decline in rates of measles transmission.

INTRODUCTION

In the pre-vaccination era in Africa measles was predominantly a disease of the young and had a devastating impact on unvaccinated populations (1). Widespread measles vaccination programmes have led to changes in transmission patterns of measles that have included increasing the average age at infection (1, 2) which has led to reduction in mortality from measles because mortality is inversely related to age at infection (3). In the city of Gweru in Zimbabwe it was observed in the late 1980s that vaccination had led to changes in epidemiology of measles. In this city vaccination against measles was commenced in 1971 and accelerated with the advent of the Expanded Programme on Immunization (EPI) in 1982-83. In 1971-89 a single dose of live hyper-attenuated Schwartz strain vaccine (0.5 mls or 1000$TCID_{50}$) was applied to children at 9 months of age. Gweru is the third largest city in Zimbabwe and has a population of 158233 (4). Measles vaccine was applied to children at 9months of age at static health facilities and no vaccination campaigns were carried out outside health facilities. This chapter reports on a study that examined the impact of this vaccination regime on measles transmission patterns and explored implications of this impact on measles control.

OUR STUDY

A retrospective observational study that used data from measles vaccination records and measles disease surveillance data related vaccination rates to dependent variables was conducted in the urban district of Gweru, Zimbabwe.

In Gweru, measles vaccinations were applied to children at eight static health facilities since 1971 and vaccination records were available since then. No vaccinations were being applied outside these health facilities. Routine vaccinations were indicated on child health cards and vaccination records/statistics were compiled monthly.

The city of Gweru had an active measles surveillance system. On this system, cases were identified on the basis of a standard clinical case definition that was available to all staff at all the city's health centres and infectious disease hospital. There were personnel that were assigned to investigate unreported infectious diseases (including measles cases) within communities (active case search). Measles case surveillance/investigation forms indicated age at infection, vaccination status, sex, presenting features of disease, whether admitted into hospital or not, treatment regime instituted, occurrence of any other cases in relation to an identified case (which would also be investigated), and outcome of illness (alive of dead). Data on vaccination status of cases was only available from 1980 and not before. Complicated cases are managed at the city's single infectious disease hospital. Data on measles cases and deaths were entered on line lists that indicated the same variables as those on case investigation forms. Data from the measles surveillance system were compiled monthly.

The main study outcome measures were; (a) Measles vaccination coverage rates, (b) Measles incidence rates, (c) Changes in age distribution of measles cases, (d) Vaccination status of measles cases, (e) Risk of contracting measles by age: age stratified measles incidence rates, (f) Rate of spread of infection in the population: age stratified cumulative proportions of measles cases.

Medians and interquartile range (IQR) were used to describe continuous non-normally distributed data. Frequencies and percentages were used to describe categorical data. Measles vaccine coverage rates were calculated by dividing the number of vaccine doses administered to those in a specified target age group by the estimated target population. Measles incidence rates were calculated as the number of notified cases per 100 000 total population. Denominators used to calculate measles incidence and vaccine coverage rates were obtained from census and inter-census data.

The Kruskal-Wallis (KW) test was used to compare medians of non-normally distributed data. Linear relationship was established using the Chi-squared test for linear trend or simple linear regression analysis, were appropriate All tests were two-sided and the cut off point for statistical significance was 5%. Data were analyzed using SPSS 20.0 for Windows.

Measles case notifications were pooled by age for the years 1967-70, 1971-83 and 1984-89. These notifications were pooled in line with three levels of measles vaccine coverage i.e., pre-vaccination (1967-70), vaccine coverage <80% (1971-83), and vaccine coverage of >80% (1984-89). From these pooled case notifications age stratified cumulative proportions of cases were determined. Three cumulative curves or plots were made from the age stratified cumulative proportions of cases. Each of the cumulative curves or plots reflected proportion of population who had experienced infection by each age group and rate of rise of this proportion was a measure of the magnitude of transmission in the population, i.e., the steeper the profile the more rapid the spread of infection in the population. These curves therefore gave an indication of the speed at which infection consumed susceptibles in various age groups.

FINDINGS

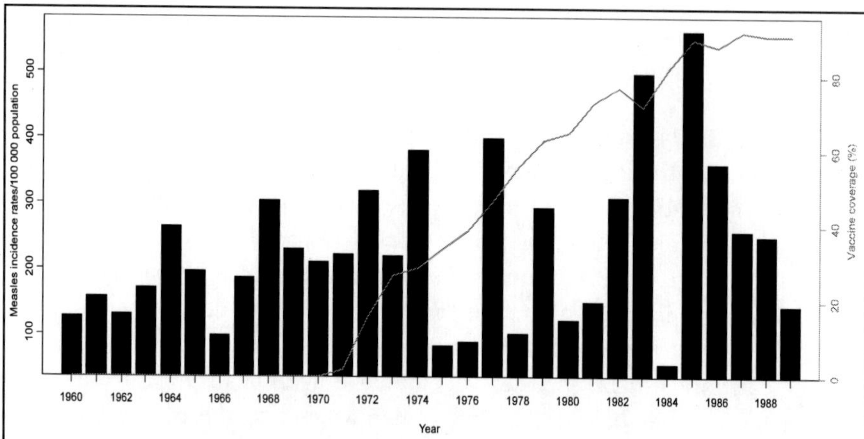

Figure 1. Measles vaccine coverage rates and measles incidence rates in Gweru city 1960-89.

Figure 1 shows measles vaccine coverage rates and measles incidence rates in Gweru city 1960-89. Vaccine coverage rates were 0% in pre-vaccination era in 1960-70 and 2 - 92% in1971-89 (Median 65, Q_1= 34, Q_3=88) when they significantly and linearly increased (χ^2 for linear trend= 567.1, $p<0.001$).

Measles incidence rates in Gweru in 1960-89 were 56.3-562.6/100 000 population (median: 215.8, Q_1=131.8, Q_3=304.9). Incidence rates in 1960-85 were 56.3- 562.6/100 000 population (median: 203.6, Q_1= 128, Q_3= 304.9) and these rates significantly linearly increased in this period (χ^2 for linear trend= 219.75, $p<0.001$) (figure 1). In 1986-89, measles incidence rates were 141.7-361.1/100 000 population (median: 253.95, Q_1= 197.4, Q_3= 309.5) and these rates significantly linearly declined (χ^2 for linear trend = 85.41, $p<0.001$). In 1960-89, measles incidence rates did not exhibit a discernable pattern of epidemics and inter-epidemic periods.

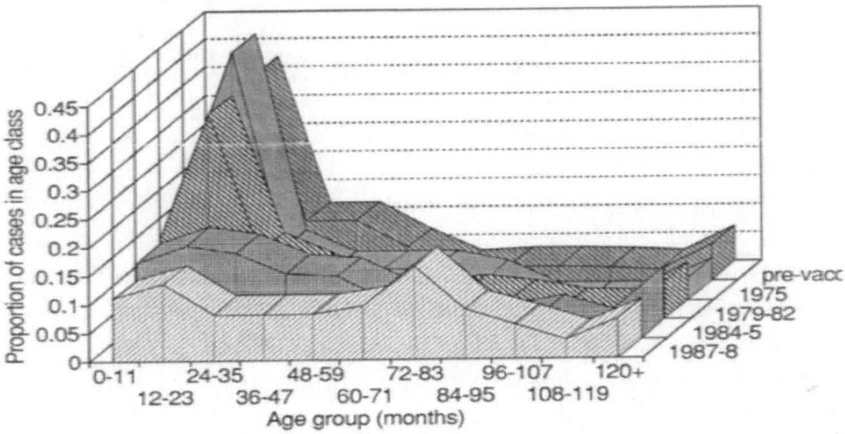

Figure 2. Measles case notifications by age in Gweru city 1967-89.

Data on measles cases that is disaggregated by age was available in Gweru since 1967and not before. Figure 2 shows distribution of measles cases reported in each age class (for selected years) in the period 1967-89. Measles notifications for the pre-vaccination period, 1967-70, were pooled. This figure illustrates detailed changes in the age distribution of measles cases that occurred in the period 1967-89. There was shift of disease from young age groups of <59 months towards older age groups of >60 months from pre-vaccination era in 1967-70 up till 1989 when vaccination coverage rates were >90%.

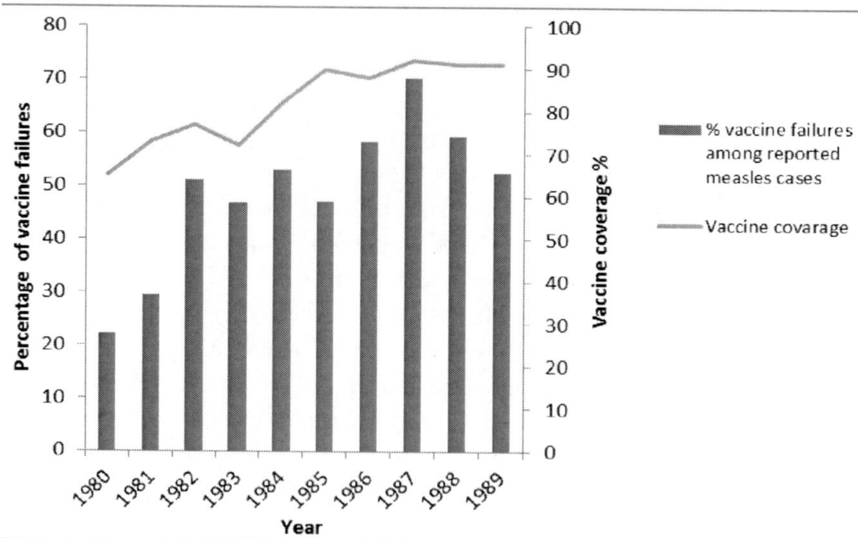

Figure 3. Measles vaccination coverage rates and percentage of vaccine failures (vaccinated cases) among all reported measles cases in Gweru city 1980-89.

Figure 3 shows v*accination status of measles cases.* Data on vaccination status of measles cases was available in Gweru since 1980. In 1980-89 among all reported measles cases 22.2-70.4% (median: 51.8, Q_1=42.6, Q_3=58.7) had had measles vaccination (vaccine failures). As vaccination coverage rates increased, the proportion of vaccine failures among all measles case notifications significantly linearly increased (Regression coefficient = 1.19, 95% CI [0.52, 1.86], Adjusted R^2=63.7%).

Proportion of vaccine failures in age group 10-59 months (among all cases reported in this age group) were not significantly different at measles vaccine coverage rates of <80% and >80% in 1980-89 (KW χ^2 = 6.01, df=1, p= 0.140) while in the same period proportion of vaccine failures in age group 60-119 months were significantly higher at vaccine coverage rates of >80% than at coverage rates of <80% (KW χ^2 = 6.55, df =1, p= 0.011). As measles vaccination coverage rates increased, proportion of vaccine failures in age group 60-119 months (among all cases reported in this age group) significantly linearly increased (Regression coefficient = 1.17, 95% CI [0.35, 1.99], Adjusted R^2= 52.1%).

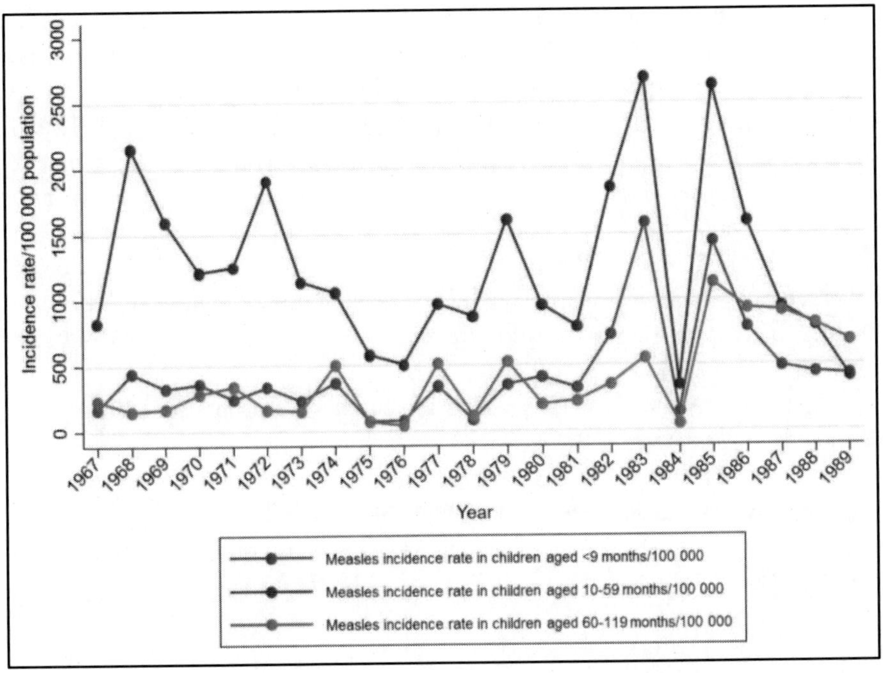

Figure 4. Measles Incidence rates in age groups <=9 months, 10-59 months and 60-119 months in Gweru City 1967-89

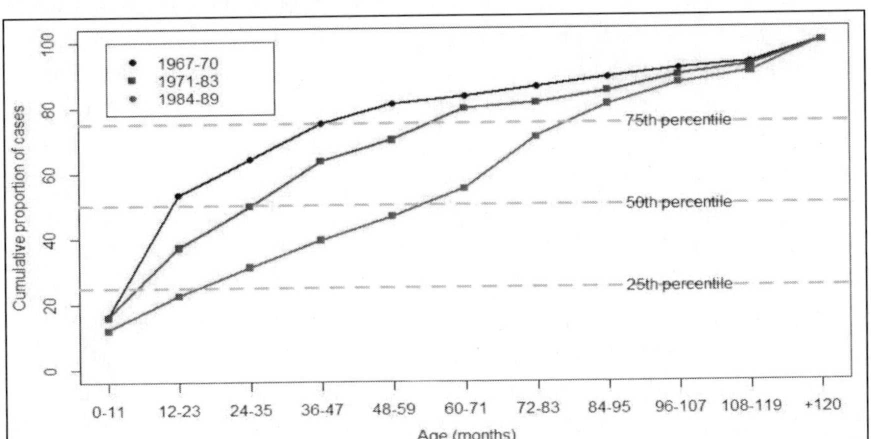

Figure 5. Cumulative proportion plots of reported measles cases for the years 1967-70 (pooled), 1971-83 (pooled) and 1984-89 (pooled) in Gweru city.

Measles incidence rates in age groups <=9, 10-59 and 60-119 months in 1967-89 are indicated in Figure 4. In pre-vaccination era and at vaccine coverage rates of <80% and >80% measles incidence rates in age group <=9 months were not significantly different (KW χ^2 = 3.65, df = 2, p= 0.161) and so were incidence rates in age group 10-59 months (KW χ^2 = 1.63, df =2, p=0.443). Measles incidence rates in age group 60-119 months in pre-vaccination era, and at vaccine coverage rates of <80 and >80% were significantly different (KW χ^2 = 6.11, df =2, p= 0.047). As measles vaccine coverage rates increased measles incidence rates in this age group significantly linearly increased (Regression coefficient = 29.88, 95% CI [13.95, 45.82], Adjusted R^2= 39.2%).

Figure 5 shows three curves which are cumulative proportions of measles cases by age for the years 1967-89.

In 1967-70, 1971-83 and 1984-89, some 75% of all reported measles cases occurred by age group 36-47 months, 48-59 months and 72-83 months respectively and thus measles transmission was most rapid in 1967-70 and least rapid in 1984-89.

DISCUSSION

The current study found that in the pre-vaccination era (1960-70), and at vaccine coverage rates of <82% (1971-85) measles incidence rates significantly increased and did not exhibit a discernible pattern of epidemics and inter-epidemic periods. It was also found that at vaccine coverage rates of >90% in 1986-89 measles incidence rates significantly declined.

Several factors could have contributed to the observed significant increase in measles incidence rates in 1960-85. Lack of vaccination in the pre-vaccination era and low measles vaccination coverage rates in 1971-83 may have sustained high measles transmission. High birth rates and population movements from rural to urban areas could have added lots of susceptibles to the urban population thus keeping transmission high (1, 5-9). Lack of a discernible pattern of epidemics and inter-epidemic periods in 1960-89 may be indicative of an unstable population growth environment where susceptibles were introduced into the urban population in big numbers. While high birth rates and migration could have ensured a continuous supply of susceptibles, densely crowded urban living conditions could have led to rapid transmission of measles (10, 11). In this study the role of (a) birth rates, (b) rural to urban population movements and (c) overcrowded living conditions in sustaining high measles transmission in Gweru were not investigated. A possible reason for the observed increase in measles incidence rates in 1960-85 could be improved disease surveillance and reporting of measles cases over the years. There is no doubt that as years progressed surveillance of communicable diseases (including measles) improved.

Measles incidence rates significantly declined in Gweru at measles vaccine coverage rates of >90% in 1986-89. This finding is very much in keeping with experiences elsewhere where sustained high vaccine coverage rates led to decline in measles transmission in communities (12-14).

In this study it was found that as vaccination coverage rates increased, proportion of vaccine failures among reported measles cases significantly increased. Occurrence of vaccine failures is blamed on a vaccine of less than 100% efficacy (15-18) or waning immunity (17-19). With a vaccine of less than 100% efficacy as vaccine coverage rates increase there would be more vaccine failures among reported cases while at lower vaccine coverage rates fewer vaccine failures are created. Increases of vaccine failures have had important public health implications in relation to measles control. Accumulation of vaccine failures in developing countries with moderate to high measles vaccine coverage rates has led to epidemics after a decline in measles transmission (18, 19). A policy issue of importance that would arise from this is that it would not be possible to either eliminate (20-22) or eradicate (23-25) measles using a strategy that would solely rely on a single application at 9 months of age of a vaccine of less than 100% efficacy as was the case in Gweru prior to 1989.

The current study found that in pre-vaccination era measles predominantly afflicted the young (<59 months age group) and as vaccine coverage rates increased the disease shifted to older children of 60-119 months of age. It was found that the shift of the disease to these older children was associated with a significant increased susceptibility (increased risk) of contracting measles by this age group compared to younger age group of <59 months. Also, it was found that as vaccine coverage rates increased there was a significant increase in occurrence of vaccine failures in this age group.

From the findings of this study, shift of disease to age group 60-119 months is likely to have arisen from increased susceptibility to contracting measles due to accumulation of vaccine failures in this age group. Explanation for accumulation of these vaccine failures among older children (and even adults) has been that for vaccine applied in infancy, vaccination of large proportion of the community reduces chances for susceptibles to be exposed to the infectious agent in infancy such that they are exposed at an older age leading to an increase in average age at infection (18, 26-29). Shift of measles transmission from younger to older age groups that is associated with accumulation vaccine failures among older age groups has occurred in some developing countries with high vaccine coverage rates of vaccine applied at 9 months of age (18, 19, 30). Measles epidemics that have occurred in communities and schools in Cape Town in South Africa (19), Swaziland (37), Jordan (30), and Harare, Zimbabwe (31) have mostly involved children who are older than 60 months of age most of whom had had vaccination. Some epidemics that have occurred among older children in schools have been associated with secondary cases in younger siblings in the community (16). In developing countries high occurrence of measles in children aged >60 months in 1989 and before was problematic in that, as a matter of policy, children were routinely only vaccinated at 9 months of age and not at an older age in that period. A public health implication of this would be that to reduce likelihood of epidemics in these susceptible older age groups there would be need to apply vaccination in these groups as a matter of policy.

Shift of disease to older children would have had implications on measles mortality. Studies from Gweru and elsewhere have shown that shift of measles in older children was protective against occurrence of complications and mortality (1, 3).

This study found that rates of transmission of measles in the population were most rapid in the pre-vaccination era particularly among the young aged <48 months with lower transmission occurring among those >48 months. The study also found that rates of measles transmission in the population declined as vaccine coverage rates increased with lowest rates of transmission experienced at vaccine coverage rates of >80%.

Studies from pre-vaccination era have shown that in densely populated communities in developing countries measles transmission was rapid and would consume mostly the underfives such that by the third birthday, three quarters of a birth cohort would have been infected and very few underfives would escape measles in childhood (32). This epidemiological picture is similar to what obtained in Gweru in the pre-vaccination era.

At vaccine coverage rates of >80%, measles transmission in the Gweru would have been curtailed by herd immunity (33-37) and this could have been particularly so after 1985 (at coverage rates >90%) when the measles vaccine coverage threshold (34, 37-39) had been breached. There are two findings from the current study that would support this observation:

a) This study found that in the period under review measles was endemic in Gweru and that measles incidence rates significantly increased from pre-vaccination era up till 1985 while at vaccine coverage rates of >90% in 1986-89 there was a significant and sustained decline in measles incidence rates.
b) At vaccine coverage rates of >80%, slightly over a third of all measles cases reported in Gweru were of age group 60-119 months. In this age group 63% of cases were vaccine failures while the remainder had not had vaccination. A likely explanation why both the vaccine failures and the unvaccinated of this age group escaped contracting measles up till this age is that they were protected by herd immunity.

In conclusion, impact of measles vaccine applied at 9 months of age on measles transmission patterns was that:

a) Measles incidence rates declined at vaccine coverage rates of >90%
b) Measles vaccine failures significantly increased as vaccine coverage rates increased
c) Age at infection shifted from age group <59 months to age group 60-119 months (as vaccine coverage rates increased) likely due to increased susceptibility of the latter age group arising from accumulation of vaccine failures in this group.
d) Rates of transmission of measles in the population declined (as vaccine coverage rates increased) likely due the fact that herd immunity retarded transmission.

Implications of this impact were that:

a. Shift of disease from the younger to older age groups meant there would be less mortality among the young.
b. Shift of disease to older children (most whom were vaccine failures) meant that there would be need to apply vaccination to this group to reduce likelihood of occurrence of epidemics in the future.

Acknowledgments

We would especially like to thank city of Gweru Public Health Department staff who helped out with extraction of data from the surveillance records and carried out data entry.

This chapter is a revised version of an original paper published in the European Journal of Preventive Medicine (Marufu T, Siziya S, Tinago W. Impact of vaccination on measles transmission patterns in Gweru city, Zimbabwe, 1960-89. Eur J Prev Med 2016;4:65-72) and the authors have obtained the permission from European Journal of Preventive Medicine to use this material.

References

[1] Goodson JL, Masresha BG, Wannemuehler K, Uzicanin A, Cochi S. Changing epidemiology of measles in Africa. J Infect Dis 2011;204(Suppl 1):S205-14.

[2] Moss WJ. Measles still has a devastating impact in unvaccinated populations. PLoS Med 2007;4:e24.

[3] Marufu T, Siziya S, Tshimanga M, Murugasampillay S, Mason E, Manyame B. Factors associated with measles complications in Gweru, Zimbabwe. East Afr Med J 2001;78:135-8.

[4] ZimStat. Census 2012. Preliminary report. Zimbabwe National Statistics Agency, Harare, Zimbabwe, 2010. URL: http://unstats.un.org/unsd/demographic/sources/census/2010_phc/Zimbabwe/ZWE_CensusPreliminary2012.pdf. Accessed 23 March 2016.

[5] Conlan AJ, Grenfell BT. Seasonality and the persistence and invasion of measles. Proc Biol Sci 2007;274:1133-41.

[6] Ferrari MJ, Grenfell BT, Strebel PM. Think globally, act locally: the role of local demographics and vaccination coverage in the dynamic response of measles infection to control. Philos Trans R Soc Lond B Biol Sci 2013;368:20120141.

[7] Earn DJ, Rohani P, Bolker BM, Grenfell BT. A simple model for complex dynamical transitions in epidemics. Science 2000;287:667-70.

[8] May RM, Anderson RM. Spatial heterogeneity and the design of immunization programs. Mathematical Biosciences 1984;72:83-111.

[9] Anderson RM, May RM. Age-related changes in the rate of disease transmission: implications for the design of vaccination programmes. J Hyg (Lond) 1985;94:365-436.

[10] Foster SO. Measles, the ultimate challenge in urban immunization In: Universal child immunization-Reaching the urban poor, Urban Examples. New York, UNICEF, 1990.

[11] Global Program for Vaccines of World Health Organization. Global measles strategy picks up pace. In: Summary of consultation on strategies to accelerate global measles control held on 27-28 April 1994; PAHO headquarters, Washington DC.

[12] Center for Disease Control and Prevention. Global measles mortality, 2000-2008. MMWR 2009;58:1321-6.

[13] Keeling MJ, Rhani P. Modelling infectious diseases in humans and animals. Princeton: Princeton University Press 2008.

[14] Goldhaber-Fiebert JD, Lipsitch M, Mahal A, Zaslavsky AM, Salomon JA. Quantifying child mortality reductions related to measles vaccination. PLoS One;2010;5:e13842.

[15] Rosenthal SR, Clements CJ. Two-dose measles vaccination schedules. Bull World Health Organ 1993;71:421-8.

[16] Marufu T, Siziya S, Tshimanga M, Xaba E, Ruwodo C, Silape Z, Baye T, Hhlazo M. Challenges posed by changes in measles transmission patterns. Cent Afr J Med 1998;44:5-8.

[17] Marufu T, Siziya S, Manyame B, Xaba E, Silape Z, Zimbizi P, Ruwodo C, Mason E, Matchaba-Hove RB, Mudyarabikwa O. Questioning the level of efficacy of the measles vaccine in use in Zimbabwe. Cent Afr J Med 1995;41:241-5.

[18] Global Programme for Vaccines and Immunization. Immunization Policy. Expanded Programme on Immunization, WHO/EPI/GEN/92.3. WHO. Geneva: WHO; 1995.

[19] Coetzee N, Hussey GD, Visser G, Barron P, Keen A. The 1992 measles epidemic in Cape Town- a changing epidemiological pattern. S Afr Med J 1994;84:145-9.

[20] de Quadros CA, Olive JM, Hersh BS, Strassburg MA, Henderson DA, Brandling-Bennett D, Alleyne GA. Measles elimination in the Americas- Evolving strategies. JAMA 1996;275:224-9.

[21] Cutts FT, Lessler J, Metcalf CJ. Measles elimination: progress, challenges and implications for rubella control. Expert Rev Vaccines 2013;12:917-32.

[22] World Health Organization. Meeting of the Strategic Advisory Group of Experts on Immunization, November 2012 - conclusions and recommendations. Wkly Epidemiol Rec 2013; 88(1):1-16.

[23] Moss WJ, Strebel P. Biological feasibility of measles eradication. J Infect Dis 2011;204(Suppl 1):S47-S53.

[24] De Quadros CA, Andrus JK, Danovaro-Holliday MC, Castillo-Solorzano C. Feasibility of global measles eradication after interruption of transmission in the Americas. Expert Rev Vaccines 2008;7:355-62.

[25] Andrus JK, de Quadros CA, Solorzano CC, Periago MR, Henderson DA. Measles and rubella eradication in the Americas Vaccine 2011;29(Suppl 4):D91-D96.

[26] Expanded Programme on Immunization. Measles control in the 1990s: Plan of action for global measles control 1992; WHO/EPI/GEN/92.3.

[27] Cutts F. Expanded Programme on Immunization-Measles control in the 1990s: Principles for the next decade, 1990; WHO/EPI/GEN/90.2.

[28] Marufu T, Siziya S. Impact of multiple dose measles vaccination on measles transmission patterns in Gweru, Zimbabwe. J Trop Pediatr 2001;47:335-8.

[29] Marufu T, Siziya S, Tinago W. Comparison of single dose and multiple dose measles vaccination strategies on measles transmission patterns. Eur J Prev Med 2015;3:80-4.

[30] Khuri-Bulos NA. Measles in Jordan: a prototype of the problems with measles in developing countries. Pediatr Infect Dis J 1995;14:22-6.

[31] Kambarami RA, Nathoo KJ, Nkrumah FK, Pirie DJ. Measles epidemic in Harare, Zimbabwe, despite high measles immunization coverage rates. Bull World Health Organ 1991;69:213-9.

[32] Morley D. Severe measles. In: Morley D, ed. Paediatric priorities in the developing world. London: Butterworths, 1979:207-30.

[33] Garnett GP. Role of herd immunity in determining the effect of vaccines against sexually transmitted disease. J Infect Dis 2005;191(Suppl 1):S97-S106.

[34] Willingham E, Helf L. What is herd immunity? URL: www.pbs.org/wgbh/nova/body/herd-immunity.html.

[35] John TJ, Samuel R. Herd immunity and herd effect: new insights and definitions. Eur J Epidemiol 2000;16:601-6.

[36] Anderson RM, May RM. Vaccination and herd immunity to infectious diseases. Nature 1985;318:323-9.

[37] Fine P, Eames K, Heymann DL. Herd immunity: A rough guide. Clin Infect Dis 2011;52:911-6.

[38] Fine PE. Herd immunity: history, theory, practice. Epidemiol Rev 1993;15:265-302.

[39] Nokes DJ, Anderson RM. Measles, mumps, and rubella vaccine: what coverage to block transmission? Lancet 1988;2:1374.

In: Measles
Editors: T. Marufu, S. Siziya et al.
ISBN: 978-1-63485-559-4

Chapter 3

CHANGES IN RATES OF MEASLES TRANSMISSION AND FORCE OF INFECTION

Tawanda Marufu[1,*], MB ChB, MSc, Willard Tinago[1], BSc, MSc, PhD and Seter Siziya[2], BA(Ed), MSc, PhD

[1]Department of Community Medicine,
University of Zimbabwe College of Health Sciences,
Harare, Zimbabwe
[2]Department of Clinical Sciences,
Copperbelt University School of Medicine, Ndola, Zambia

A study compared rates of measles transmission and force of infection in pre-vaccination era (1967), and at measles vaccine coverage rates of 50-80% (1978-84) and >90% (1989).Using measles surveillance data cumulative proportions of measles cases by age were determined for the years 1967, 1978-89 (pooled) and 1989. From the cumulative curves estimates of the age dependent rate of infection with measles (force of infection) was determined for the years 1967, 1978-84 and 1989. In 1967 and 1978-84 some 75% of all measles cases occurred by age group 36-47 months while in 1989 this occurred by age group 72-83 months thus measles transmission was most rapid in 1967 and least rapid in 1989. Variation of force of infection between years 1967, 1978-84 and 1967

* Correspondence: Tawanda Marufu, University of Zimbabwe College of Health Sciences, Box A 178, Avondale, Harare, Zimbabwe. E-mail: marufut@yahoo.com.

showed that force of infection was not significantly different between the years for age groups 24-35, 36-47 and 48-59 months. Meanwhile, the force of infection varied between the years in the rest of the age groups, with a significant reduction in force of infection over the years for age groups <11, and 12-23 months; and significant increases in force of infection were observed in the age groups 60-71, 72-83, 84-95, 96-107 and 108-119 months. Measles transmission rates in the community were highest in pre-vaccination era and least at vaccination coverage rates of >90% most likely due to effect of herd immunity. From pre-vaccination era (1967) to vaccine coverage rates of >90% (1989) there was a shift in force of infection from young age groups <23 months to older age groups of 60-119 months most likely due to accumulation of susceptibles in these older age groups. Shift in force of infection to older age groups would have been responsible for the shift in age at infection to these older age groups.

INTRODUCTION

Measles is a major cause of morbidity and mortality in developing countries (1). High measles vaccine coverage rates have reduced disease, disability and death attributed to measles (2). Over and above the reduction in measles morbidity and mortality, in developing countries widespread measles vaccination has led to changes in measles epidemiology that have included changes in transmission patterns and force of infection (3). A study was carried out in the city of Gweru in Zimbabwe to investigate changes in measles transmission rates and force of infection from the pre-vaccination era in 1967 to 1989 when measles vaccine coverage rates (for the vaccine applied at 9 months at age) were >90%.

OUR STUDY

A retrospective observational study used data from measles vaccination records and measles disease surveillance data. Rates of measles transmission in the community and force of infection were determined for the years 1967 (pre-vaccination period), 1978-84 (when vaccine coverage rates were 50-80%) and 1989 (when vaccine coverage rates were >90%).

In Gweru, measles vaccinations were applied to children at static health facilities since 1971 and vaccination records were available since then.

Routine vaccinations were indicated on child health cards and vaccination records/statistics were compiled monthly.

The city of Gweru had an active measles surveillance system. On this system, cases were identified on the basis of a standard clinical case definition that was available to all staff at all the city's health centres and infectious disease hospital. There were personnel that were assigned to investigate unreported infectious diseases (including measles cases) within communities (active case search). Measles case surveillance/investigation forms indicated age at infection, vaccination status, sex, presenting features of disease, whether admitted into hospital or not, treatment regime instituted, occurrence of any other cases in relation to an identified case (which would also be investigated), and outcome of illness (alive of dead). Data on vaccination status of cases was only available from 1980 and not before. Complicated cases were managed at the city's single infectious disease hospital. Data on measles cases and deaths were entered on line lists that indicated the same variables as those on case investigation forms. Data from the measles surveillance system were compiled monthly.

Cumulative proportions of measles cases by age were determined for the years 1967, 1978-89 (pooled) and 1989. Because the cumulative proportion curves were well age-stratified an estimate of the age-dependent rate of infection with measles (force of infection) was determined for the years 1967, 1978-84 (pooled) and 1989 from these curves using methodology described by Grenfell and Anderson (4).

The main outcome measures were: (a) Measles vaccination coverage rates for the years 1967, 1978-84 and 1989, (b) Rates of measles transmission in the population in the 1967, 1978-84 and 1989 and (c) Force of infection in the years 1967, 1978-84 and 1989.

FINDINGS

Vaccine coverage rates were 0% in pre-vaccination era in 1967 and >92% in 1989. In1978-84 vaccine coverage rates were 50-80% (median: 72, $Q_1 = 63$, $Q_3=77$).

Figure 1 shows three curves which are cumulative proportions of measles cases by age for the years 1967, 1978-84 (pooled) and 1989. In this study each of the cumulative curves or plots indicates proportion of population who have experienced infection by each age group and rate of rise of this proportion is a measure of the magnitude of transmission in the population or community i.e., the steeper the profile the more rapid the spread of infection in the population. These curves therefore give an indication of the speed at which infection consumed susceptibles in various age groups.

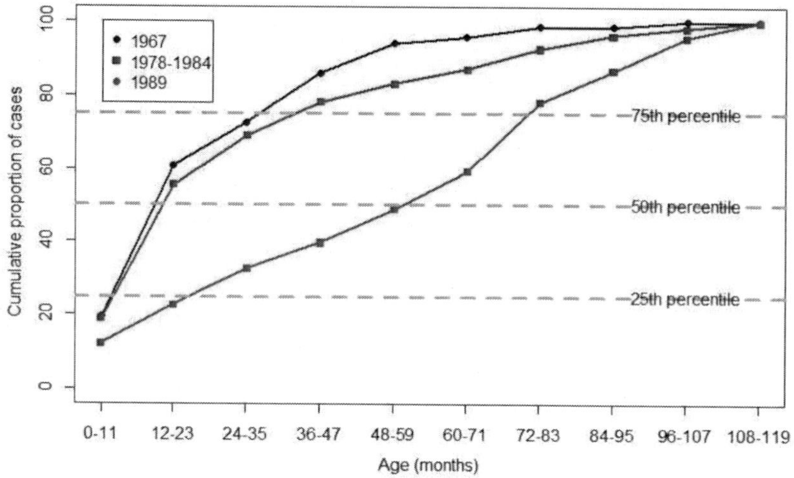

Figure 1. Cumulative proportion plots of reported measles cases for the years 1967, 1978-84 (pooled) and 1989.

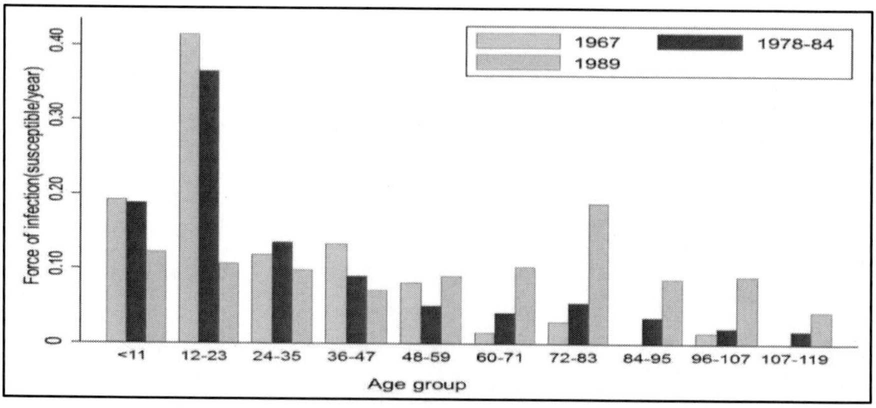

Figure 2. Age stratified rate of infection (force of infection) for the years 1967, 1978-84 (pooled) and 1989.

In 1967 and 1978-84 some 75% of all reported measles cases occurred by age group 36-47 months while in 1989 this occurred by age group 72-83 months, meaning that rapidity of measles transmission was steepest in 1967 and least steep in 1989.

Table 1. Variation in force of infection between the years 1967, 1978-84 (pooled) and 1989 and trends in force of infection in 1967-89

	Force of infection in years				
Age groups in months	1967	1978-84	1989	Variation in force of infection between the years 1967, 1978-84 and 1989: χ^2 (p-value)	Trends in force of infection between 1967 and 1989: χ^2 for trend (p-value)
<11	0.19	0.18.	0.12	6.20 (0.045)	4.56 (0.033)
12-23	0.42	0.37	0.11	66.31 (<0.001)	54.13 (<0.001)
24-35	0.12	0.14	0.09	2.42 (0.298)	0.84 (0.360)
36-47	0.13	0.09	0.07	4.17 (0.124)	3.77 (0.052)
48-59	0.08	0.05	0.09	5.91 (0.052)	0.89 (0.346)
60-71	0.02	0.04	0.10	18.71 (<0.001)	17.20 (<0.001)
72-83	0.03	0.06	0.19	50.68 (<0.001)	41.24 (<0.001)
84-95	0.0	0.04	0.09	18.85 (<0.001)	18.48 (<0.001)
96-107	0.02	0.02	0.09	28.79 (<0.001)	21.53 (<0.001)
108-119	0.0	0.02	0.04	9.22 (0.010)	9.04 (0.003)

Table 1 and Figure 2 show age stratified rate of infection which is an indication of the likelihood of a susceptible being infected per unit time in each age group. Highest force of infection occurred in age group <23 months in 1967. From age group 24-35 months susceptibility to infection by age declined up till age 60-71 months when force of infection petered off. In 1989 highest force of infection was in age group 60-83 months with a peak in age group 72-83 months.

In 1978-84 force of infection in age groups <59 months was something of a mirror image of susceptibility experienced in 1967 but unlike in 1967 in age groups 60-119 months there was an increase in susceptibility to infection.

Table 1 shows variation in force of infection between the years 1967, 1978-84 and 1989. It also shows trends in force of infection between 1967 and 1989. Force of infection was not significantly different between the years for age groups 24-35, 36-47 and 48-59 months. Meanwhile, the force of infection varied between the years in the rest of the age groups, with a significant reduction in force of infection over the years for age groups <11, and 12-23 months; and significant increases in force of infection were observed in the age groups 60-71, 72-83, 84-95, 96-107 and 108-119 months.

DISCUSSION

This study found that rates of transmission of measles in the population were most rapid in the pre-vaccination era (and also at vaccine coverage rates of <80%) particularly among the young aged <48 months with little transmission occurring among those >48 months.

Studies from pre-vaccination era have shown that in densely populated communities in developing countries measles transmission was rapid and would consume mostly the underfives such that by the third birthday three quarters of a birth cohort would have been infected and very few underfives would escape measles in childhood (5). This epidemiological picture is similar to what obtained in Gweru in the pre-vaccination era.

The current study found that rates of measles transmission in the population declined as vaccine coverage rates increased with lowest rates of transmission experienced at vaccine coverage rates of > 90%. At vaccine coverage rates of >90% measles transmission in the Gweru would have been retarded by herd immunity [6-10] and this could have been particularly so after measles vaccine coverage threshold (6, 11-13) had been breached.

This study found that force of infection was highest in children aged <23 months (with a peak in 12-23 months) in pre-vaccination era and at vaccine coverage rates of <80%. It was also found that in age group <23 months force of infection significantly declined in 1967-89.

A high force of infection in children aged <23 months found in the current study is in keeping with the observation that in developing countries in pre-vaccination era measles was predominantly a disease of the very young who would be susceptible to infection after loss of transplacentally acquired maternal antibodies (5). Unlike findings of the current study, in developed countries such as USA and UK in the pre-vaccination era peak of force of infection was highest in children aged 5-9 years (5, 14).

Decline in force of infection in children aged <23 months in 19667-89 observed in the current study would have been due to improved levels of immunity in this age group arising from continuous application of vaccine to successive 9 month old cohorts (from the time vaccination was commenced in 1971) and the high vaccine coverage rates of >90% that had been attained among these cohorts by 1989.

The current study found that in 1989 highest force of infection was in children aged 60-119 months (with a peak in age group 72-83 months) and that the force of infection in this age group had significantly risen in 1967-89. A study that investigated susceptibility to measles infection in children aged

10-119 months in the city of Gweru in Zimbabwe in 1988 (15) had findings that were similar to those of the current study. That study (15) found that children in older age groups were more susceptible to infection than those in younger age groups and this was blamed on accumulation of vaccine failures (in these older age groups) arising from a vaccine of less than 100% efficacy. Shift of measles transmission from younger to older age groups that is associated with accumulation of vaccine failures among older age groups has occurred in some developing countries with high vaccine coverage rates of measles vaccine applied at 9 months of age (16-18). A plausible explanation for the change in age at infection from younger to older age groups would be that accumulation of vaccine failures led to an increase in force of infection. It is most likely that increase in force of infection in older age groups found in the current study in years 1978-84 and 1989 would have arisen from a similar experience.

In conclusion, measles transmission rates in the community were highest in pre-vaccination era and least at vaccination coverage rates of >90% most likely due to effect of herd immunity. From pre-vaccination era (1967) to vaccine coverage rates of >90% (1989) there was a shift in force of infection from young age groups <23 months to older age groups of 60-119 months most likely due to accumulation of susceptibles in these older age groups. Shift in force of infection to older age groups would have been responsible for the shift in age at infection to these older age groups.

ACKNOWLEDGMENTS

We would especially like to thank city of Gweru Public Health Department staff who helped out with extraction of data from the surveillance records and carried out data entry.

This chapter is a revised version of an original paper published in the European Journal of Preventive Medicine (Marufu T, Tinago W, Siziya S. Changes in Rates of Measles Transmission and Force of Infection in Gweru City, Zimbabwe: A Retrospective Study. European Journal of Preventive Medicine 2016;4:28-31) and the authors have obtained the permission from European Journal of Preventive Medicine to use this material.

REFERENCES

[1] Moss WJ. Measles still has a devastating impact in unvaccinated populations. PLoS Med 2007;4:e24.

[2] Andre FE, Booy R, Bock HL, Clemens J, Datta SK, John TJ, Lee W, et al. Vaccination greatly reduces disease, disability, death and inequality worldwide. Bull World Health Organ 2008;86:81-160.

[3] Goodson JL, Masresha BG, Wannemuehler K, Uzicanin A, Cochi S. Changing epidemiology of measles in Africa. J Infect Dis 2011;204(Suppl 1):S205-S214.

[4] Grenfell BT, Anderson RM. The estimation of age related rates of infection from case notifications and serological data. J Hyg Camb 1985;95:419-36.

[5] Morley D. Severe measles. In: Morley D, ed. Paediatric priorities in the developing world. London: Butterworths, 1979:207-30.

[6] Willingham E, Helft L. What is herd immunity? URL: www.pbs.org/wgbh/nova/body/herd-immunity.html

[7] Garnnet GP. Role of herd immunity in determining the effect of vaccines against sexually transmitted disease J Infect Dis 2005;191(Suppl 1):S97-S106.

[8] John TJ, Samuel R. Herd immunity and herd effect: new insights and definitions. Eur J Epidemiol 2000;16:601-6.

[9] Anderson RM, May RM. Vaccination and herd immunity to infectious diseases. Nature, 1985;318:323-9.

[10] Anderson RM, May RM. Infectious diseases of humans: dynamics and control. Oxford: Oxford University Press, 1991.

[11] Fine P, Eames K, Heymann DL. "Herd Immunity": A rough guide. Clin Infect Dis 2011;52:911-6.

[12] Fine PEM. Herd immunity: History, theory, practice. Epidemiol Rev 1993;15:265-302.

[13] Nokes DJ, Anderson RM. Measles, mumps and rubella vaccine: what coverage to block transmission? Lancet 1988;2:1374.

[14] Centers for Disease Control and Prevention. Measles. In: Pink Book. Epidemiology and prevention of vaccine-preventable diseases, 13th Edition. Atlanta, GA: CDC, 1995:209-29.

[15] Marufu T, Murugasampillay S, Siziya S, Manyame B, Silape-Marufu Z, Xaba E, Zimbizi P, Ruwodo C, Mudyarabikwa O. Is the protection afforded vaccinees the same in children of all age groups? Cent Afr J Med 1995;41:144-7.

[16] Global Programme for Vaccines and Immunization. Immunization policy. Expanded programme on immunization. Geneva: WHO/EPI/GEN/92.3, 1995.

[17] Coetzee N, Hussey GD, Visser G, Barron P, Keen A. The 1992 measles epidemic in Cape Town-a changing epidemiological pattern S Afr Med J 1994;84:145-9.

[18] Khuri-Bulos NA. Measles in Jordan: a prototype of the problems with measles in developing countries. Pediatr Infect Dis J 1995;14:22-6.

In: Measles
Editors: T. Marufu, S. Siziya et al.
ISBN: 978-1-63485-559-4

Chapter 4

CHALLENGES POSED BY CHANGES IN MEASLES TRANSMISSION PATTERNS

Tawanda Marufu[1,*], MB ChB, MSc, Seter Siziya[1], BA (Ed), MSc, PhD, Mufuta Tshimanga[1], MD, MPH, Elizabeth Xaba[2], MD, MSc, Chris Ruwodo[2], MSc, Zenzo Silape[2], BA, Tsitsi Baye[2] and Melisa Hhlazo[2]

[1]Department of Community Medicine,
University of Zimbabwe Medical School, Harare, Zimbabwe
[2]Public Health Department, City of Gweru, Gweru, Zimbabwe

The objective of the study was to quantify changes in measles transmission patterns. All measles cases identified in 1998 in the measles surveillance data were analyzed. Main outcome measures were: Proportion of cases in age group 60-119 months, proportions of vaccinated and unvaccinated cases in age group 60-119 months, and occurrence of cases in schools. Measles vaccination coverage was 91%. Incidence rate of measles was 205 per 100,000 population. The age group 60-119 months accounted for 49% of all reported cases and 68% of cases in this age group were vaccinated. There were measles epidemics in

* Correspondence: Tawanda Marufu, University of Zimbabwe College of Health Sciences, Box A 178, Avondale, Harare, Zimbabwe. E-mail: marufut@yahoo.com.

schools and these were associated with occurrence of secondary cases in younger siblings in the community. Case fatality rate and mortality rate were 0.4% and one per 100,000 population respectively. High measles transmission in children of school going age could spill into the community through generation of secondary cases among younger siblings and this could result in high morbidity and mortality in this vulnerable group. It is recommended that either revaccination at school entry or mass vaccination campaigns be carried out in affected age groups at schools to reduce occurrence of epidemics.

INTRODUCTION

Measles is a highly visible and important disease in developing countries, causing 1.4 to 1.8 million deaths annually (1, 2). In recent years the epidemiology of measles has been changing in developing countries on account of vaccination (3).

The city of Gweru, Zimbabwe, has a population of 124,735 (1992 census). In this city measles vaccination has been the main strategy of measles control. Measles vaccine (0.5 mls or 1,000 $TCID_{50}$ of hyper-attenuated Schwarz strain vaccine) is applied to children at nine months of age from static health facilities. Under this vaccination regime the epidemiology of measles has been changing. This chapter reports on a study which looked at the epidemiology of measles in Gweru in 1988 in order to quantify changes in measles transmission patterns.

OUR STUDY

Measles surveillance data that was collected prospectively in 1998 was analyzed. In Gweru measles cases were identified on the basis of a standard case definition which was available to staff at all primary health care facilities and the city's infectious disease hospital. There were personnel who were assigned to investigate occurrence of unreported infectious diseases (including measles cases) within communities (active case search). Measles surveillance forms which were in use indicated age at infection, gender, vaccination status, presenting features of disease, need for hospitalization or lack of it, treatment regime, outcome of illness (alive or dead) and occurrence of any other cases in relation to an identified case (which would also be investigated). Measles data for this study arose from this surveillance system.

All measles cases and deaths identified through both passive and active surveillance in 1988 were included in the study.

A cross sectional vaccine coverage survey was conducted in children aged 10-23 months in Gweru in 1988 and thus the vaccination coverage rate indicated in the results section of this study arose from this survey.

Disease investigation reports and surveillance data were reviewed. From these the following were determined: occurrence of cases by month in 1988, incidence rate, case fatality/mortality rate, occurrence of complications among cases, proportions of cases in each age group in ages zero to 120+ months, proportions of vaccinated and unvaccinated cases in each age group in ages 10-119 months and occurrence of cases in schools.

FINDINGS

Of the 450 children aged 10 to 23 months who were included in the cross sectional vaccination survey in 1988, 409 (91%) were vaccinated. Of the 409 children who were vaccinated, 401 had documentary proof of that vaccination on the child health cards. Eight did not have such cards but their guardians were positive that they had had measles vaccination.

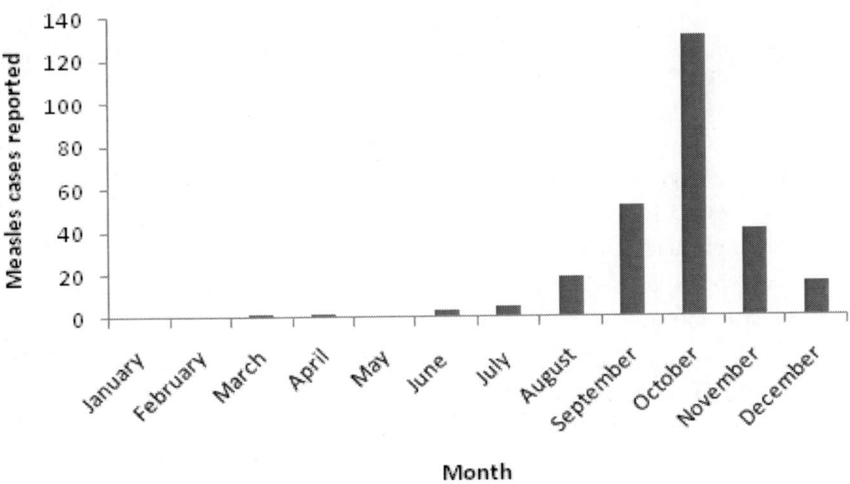

Figure 1. Occurrence of measles cases in Gweru, January to December, 1988.

Figure 1 shows cases reported in each month of 1988 in Gweru. Two hundred and seventy one cases were reported in 1988 and this represented a morbidity rate of 205 per 100 000 population in that year. Of the 271 cases, 12 (4%) occurred between January and July. From August the number of reported cases started increasing. The highest number of cases was reported in October when 131 (48%) cases were reported. After October cases declined.

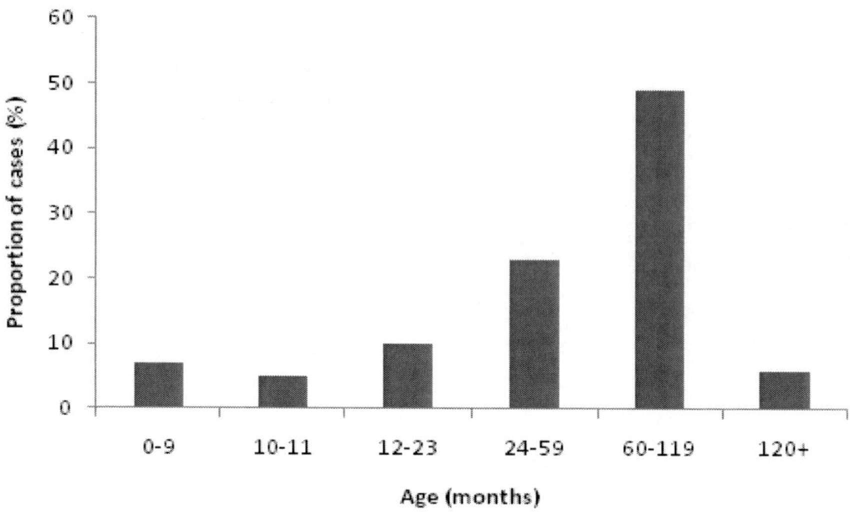

Figure 2. Proportions of reported cases in each age group in ages zero to 120+ months in Gweru in 1988.

Figure 2 shows proportions of cases reported in ages zero to 120+ months in 1988. Cases aged 0-9 months and 10-11 months accounted for 7% and 5% of cases reported in 1988, respectively. Of the 271 cases reported in 1988, cases in age groups 12-23, 24-59 and 60-119 months accounted for 10%, 23% and 49% respectively; while the age group 120+ months accounted for 6% of reported cases.

Figure 3 shows proportions of vaccinated and unvaccinated cases in ages 10 -119 months. In age groups 10-11, 12-23, 24-59 and 60-119 months, 63 to 68% of cases were vaccinated.

In 1988, 183 cases were reported in September to October which was the beginning of the school term. Ninety seven of the 183 cases were in the first or second year of elementary school (Grades 1 and 2) and on the case investigation forms they gave a history of having had a classmate with measles prior to them developing a similar condition. In the same period 56 children aged <5 years had a history of having developed measles after an elder sister or brother (whose history of disease was associated with transmission in school) had had a similar condition. Figure 4 shows an epidemic curve drawn for St Paul's Primary School in Gweru where an epidemic involving 18 pupils was investigated in September 1988. One grade 1 pupil aged six years (the only case that died in 1988) from this school died of measles associated complications during acute illness.

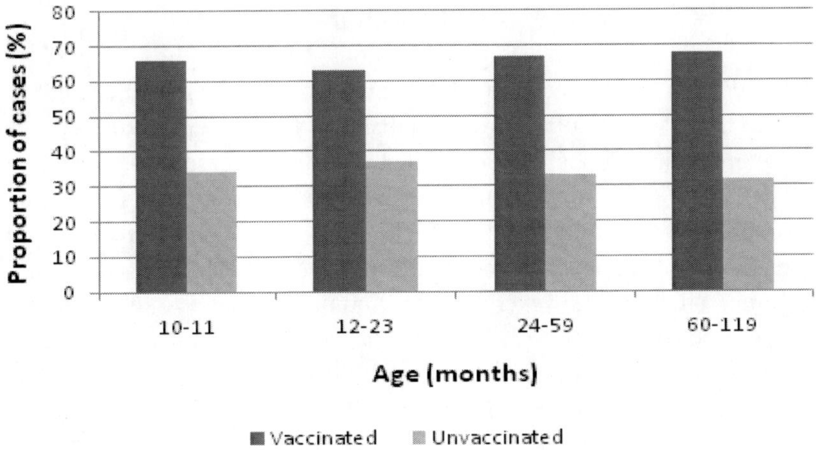

Figure 3. Proportions of vaccinated and unvaccinated cases in each age group for ages 10 to 119 months in Gweru in 1988.

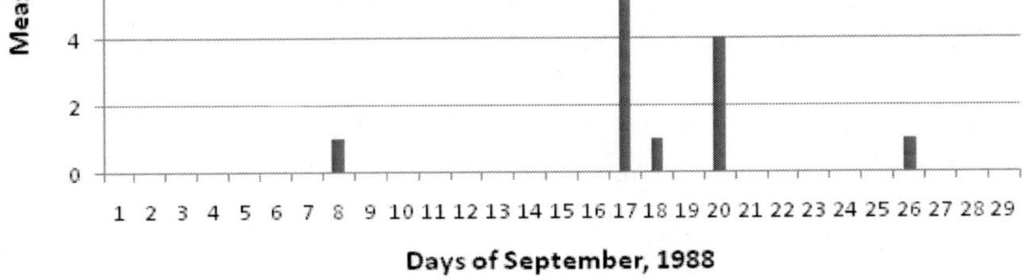

Figure 4. Measles epidemic curve for St Paul's Primary School in Gweru in September 1988.

In 1988, of the 271 measles cases, 59 (22%) had measles complications. These complications included diarrhea (39 cases), pneumonia (13 cases), laryngo-tracheo-bronchitis or coup (one case), tonsillitis (three cases) and malnutrition (three cases). As indicated earlier, one case died (of croup) in 1988, representing a case fatality rate of 0.4% and mortality rate of one per 100 000 population.

DISCUSSION

In 1988, 7% of cases occurred under nine months of age. This finding is similar to that of other studies from Zimbabwe (4,5). An epidemic study from the City of Harare, Zimbabwe, found that out of 4357 cases, 485 (11%) were under the age of nine months (4), while an epidemic report from Chimanimani in rural Zimbabwe found that out of 102 cases, four (4%) were aged under nine months (5). The level of occurrence of cases <9 months of age found in the current study is, however, unlike findings of studies (6) from other developing countries were 20% to 30% of cases occur in this group. Large cities in Africa have reported high morbidity and mortality in infants <9 months of age (7). These cities include Kinshasa in Zaire (8), Niamey in Niger (9) and Maputo in Mozambique (10).

Occurrence of a high proportion of measles aged <9 months is said to be associated with early loss of transplacentally obtained maternal antibodies (11). Vaccine efficacies of 84-91% and 86- 94% found in studies from Maputo (9) and Niamey (10) respectively would seem to suggest that at the time of vaccination most children would have lost maternal antibodies. Studies from Harare (4) and Gweru (12) found vaccine efficacies of 73-81% and 73% respectively, suggesting (11) that at the time of vaccination 20-30% of children still have maternal antibodies. Thus the low levels of vaccine efficacy found in Harare and Gweru may be suggestive of late loss of maternal antibodies and hence the low occurrence of cases under nine months of age in these cities.

The current study found that found that in 1988 most cases occurred in the age group 60-119 months. This finding concurs with those of studies from developing countries or areas with medium to high vaccine coverage rates where a shift in measles transmission from young age groups to older age groups has been observed (13). In Swaziland (14), Lesotho (14), Jordan (15) and Botswana (16), 41 to 62% of measles cases attended to at health facilities were in children aged five years and older. Like in Gweru, in Swaziland (14),

Lesotho (14) and Cape Town in South Africa (17) the shift of disease to older age groups has led to measles epidemics in schools.

In this study it was found that some children who contracted measles in school infected younger siblings at home. A study from Burundi had similar findings. That study found that school children were an important source of infection for young siblings (18). There have been concerns that outbreaks of measles in school age children could lead to infection among younger children, resulting in untoward consequences that include high case fatality rates in the younger cases (14).

In 1988 in Gweru at vaccination coverage rates of 91%, the proportion of vaccinated cases was higher than that of unvaccinated cases. This is an expected result of high coverage (3) since the measles vaccine that was in use was less than 100% efficacy (19). It is said that this increase in the proportion of vaccinated cases is relative and not an increase in the absolute number of cases among children previously immunized (3). In the current study this would be true for age groups 10-23 and 24-59 months where the increase in the proportion of vaccinated cases was accompanied by a low occurrence of cases in these age groups. However, the same cannot be said for the age group 60-119 months where an increase in the proportion of cases, arising from the shift of disease to this age group, was accompanied by an increase in the proportion of vaccinated cases in the same age group.

The shift of disease from young to older age groups (as observed in the current study) is said to be an expected occurrence at high vaccine coverage rates in programmes that concentrate on application of vaccine in children under one year of age (14,18). The explanation given for this has been that programs that vaccinate a portion of the birth cohort slow down the rate of entry of new susceptibles into the population thus leaving some children susceptible to infection till an older age, leading to a shift in age distribution of measles towards older children (18). The basis for this explanation is that the children who would get the disease when they are older would be those that were not immunized when they were young but missed getting infected then. Now, because young cohorts are better protected on account of high vaccination coverage, the disease shifts to these susceptible older children (14). Thus, according to this explanation, the shift of disease would arise from an accumulation of unvaccinated cases. This contradicts findings of the current study in that 68% of cases in age group 60-119 months were vaccinated. Thus in this case, the shift of the disease to older age groups represents an accumulation of susceptible vaccinated cases (vaccine failures) and not unvaccinated cases. This finding concurs with that of another study from

Gweru (20). That study, which looked at the protection afforded vaccinees in different age groups, found that vaccinated children in older age groups had the same risk of contracting measles as the unvaccinated while in young age groups (under five years) risk of contracting measles was higher in unvaccinated than vaccinated children. The study concluded that the shift of disease to older age groups is an accumulation of vaccine failures. A study from Jordan (15) has made similar observations. Accumulation of vaccine failures in older age groups (as found in current study) has played an important role in measles transmission. Epidemics which have occurred in communities or schools in Harare in Zimbabwe (4), Swaziland (14), Jordan (15) and Cape Town in South Africa (17) have mostly involved children who are older than 60 months of age and most of whom were vaccinated.

In the current study it was found that measles mortality was low. This finding is similar to what has been observed elsewhere (15). Measles mortality has been declining worldwide (2). Reasons indicated for this decline have included improved care of complicated cases (2,21) and vaccination (18). A study from Gweru has shown that improved care of complicated cases has played an important role in the decline of measles mortality in this city (22). Studies from other developing countries have found that vaccination reduces measles mortality through increases in age at infection (13,23) and leads to less severe infection for vaccinated cases (23,25). It could well be that in Gweru, where the disease shifted to older age groups and the proportion of vaccinated cases increased, similar mechanisms were at play in the reduction in measles mortality observed in the current study.

In conclusion, this study found that measles shifted to older age groups of 60-119 months, most of who were vaccinated, and accompanied by occurrences of epidemics in schools. There was evidence that measles contracted at school by school aged children could spill into the community through generation of secondary cases among younger siblings at home. Because measles transmission mostly occurred among an age group for which vaccination was not ordinarily provided, there is the need for a rethink on the vaccination policy. Policy options that could be explored include revaccination of children at school entry or mounting vaccination campaigns in the affected age groups periodically in schools, the timing of which would be such that vaccine failures would not accumulate to a point where epidemics would occur.

ACKNOWLEDGMENTS

This chapter is a revised version of an original paper published in the Central African Journal of Medicine (Marufu T, Siziya S, Tshimanga M, Xaba E, Ruwodo C, Silape Z, Baye T, Hhlazo M. Challenges posed by changes in measles transmission patterns. Central African Journal of Medicine 1998;44:5-8) and the authors have obtained the permission from Central African Journal of Medicine to use this material.

REFERENCES

[1] Karzon DT. Control of acute lower respiratory illness in the developing world: an assessment of vaccine intervention. Rev Infect Dis 1991;13(Suppl 6):S571-7.

[2] Expanded Programme on Immunization. Measles control-a global battle in progress: Recommendations for remainder of the decade. EPI Update Febr 1993.

[3] Expanded Programme on Immunization Measles control in the 1990s: Plan of action for global measles control. Geneva: WHO, WHO/EPI/GEN/92.3, 1992.

[4] Kambarami RA, Nathoo KJ, Nkrumah FK, Pirie DJ. Measles epidemic in Harare, Zimbabwe, despite high measles immunization coverage rates. Bull World Health Organ 1991;69:213-9.

[5] Tumwine JK. Measles in Chimanimani, Zimbabwe. E Afr Med J 1989;66:531-4.

[6] Markowtz LE, Orenstein WA. Measles vaccines. Pediatr Clin North Am 1990;37:603-25.

[7] Cutts FT. Immunological basis for immunization No.7: Measles. Geneva: WHO, WHO/EPI/GEN/93.17, 1993.

[8] Cutts FT. Strategies to improve immunization services in urban Africa. Bull World Health Organ 1991;69:407-13.

[9] Malfait P, Jataou IM, Jollet MC, Margot A, De Benoist AC, Moren A. Measles epidemic in urban community of Niamey: Transmission patterns, vaccine efficacy and immunization strategies, Niger, 1990 to 1991. Pediatr Infect Dis J 1994;13:38-44.

[10] Cutts FT, Monteiro O, Tabard P, Cliff J. Measles control in Maputo, Mozambique, using a single dose Schwarz vaccine at age nine months. Bull World Health Organ 1994;72:227-31.

[11] Foster OS, McFraland DA, John AM. Measles. In: Jamison DT, Mosley WH, Measham AR, Bobadilla JL, eds. Disease control priorities in developing countries. Oxford: World Bank, Oxford Medical Publications,1993:161-87.

[12] Marufu T, Siziya S, Manyame B, Xaba E, Silape-Marufu Z, Zimbizi P, Ruwodo C, Mason E, Matchaba-Hove RB, Mudyarabikwa O. Questioning the level of efficacy of the measles vaccine in use in Zimbabwe. Cent Afr J Med 1995;41:241-4.

[13] Global Programme for Vaccines and Immunization. Immunization Policy. Geneva: WHO/EPI/GEN/95.3, 1995.

[14] Cutts FT. Measles control in the 1990s: principles for the next Decade. Geneva: WHO/EPI/GEN 90.2, 1990.

[15] Khuri-Bhulos NA. Measles in Jordan: a prototype of the problems with measles in developing countries. Pediatr Infect Dis J 1995;14:22-6.

[16] Davis R Revised measles agenda for the 1990s: from control to pre-eradication. Int Child Health 1991;II:45-50.

[17] Coetzee N, Hussey GD, Visser G Baron P, Keen A. The 1992 measles epidemic in Cape Town - A changing epidemiological pattern. S Afr Med J 1994;84:145-6.

[18] Cutts FT, Henderson RH, Clements CJ, Chen RT, Patriarca PA. Principles of measles control. Bull World Health Organ 1991;69:1-7.

[19] Rosenthal SR, Clements CJ. Two dose measles vaccination schedules. Bull World Health Organ 1993;71:421-8.

[20] Marufu T, Murugasampillay S, Siziya S, Manyame B, Silape-Marufu Z, Xaba E, et al. Is the protection afforded measles vaccinees the same in children of all age group? Cent Afr J Med 1995;41:144-7.

[21] Division of Diarrhoeal and acute respiratory disease control, global programme for vaccines and immunization and expanded programme on immunization. Clinical research on the treatment of measles: report of a meeting. Banjul, Gambia, 3-5 November 1993. Geneva: WHO/ CDR/95.15 and WHO/EPI/GEN/95.07, 1995.

[22] Marufu T, Siziya S, Murugasampillay S, Mason E, Manyame B, Tshimanga M. Measles complications: the importance of their management in reducing mortality attributed to measles. Cent Afr J Med 1997;43:162-5.

[23] Samb B, Aaby P, Whittle H, Seck AMC, Simondon F. Decline in measles case fatality ratio after introduction of measles immunization in rural Senegal. Am J Epidemiol 1997;145:51-7.

[24] Aaby P, Bukh J, Leeroy J, Lisse MI, Mordhorst CH, Pedersen IR. Vaccinated children get milder measles infection: a community study from Guinea-Bissau. J Infect Dis 1986;154:858-63.

[25] Oshitani H, Mpabalwani M, Kasolo F, Mizuta K, Luo NP, Bhat GJ,Suzuki H, Numazaki Y. Measles infection in hospitalized children in Lusaka, Zambia. Ann Trop Paediatr 1995; 15:167-72.

In: Measles
Editors: T. Marufu, S. Siziya et al.

ISBN: 978-1-63485-559-4

Chapter 5

QUESTIONING THE LEVEL OF EFFICACY OF THE MEASLES VACCINE IN USE IN ZIMBABWE

Tawanda Marufu[1,*], MB ChB, MSc,
Seter Siziya[1], BA (Ed), MSc, PhD,
Boniface Manyame, MB ChB, MPH[2],
Elizabeth Xaba[3], MD, MSc,
Zenzo Silape[3], BA, Perpetua Zimbizi[3], BSc,
Chris Ruwodo[3], MSc, Elizabeth Mason[4], MB ChB, MSc,
Reginald B Matchaba-Hove[1], MB ChB, MSc
and Oliver Mudyarabikwa[1], BA, MSc, PhD

[1]Department of Community Medicine,
University of Zimbabwe Medical School, Harare, Zimbabwe
[2]UNICEF Zimbabwe Country Office, Harare, Zimbabwe
[3]City of Gweru Health Department, Gweru, Zimbabwe
[4]WHO Country Office, Harare, Zimbabwe

A prospective study was carried out between 1987 and 1989 in the city of Gweru (Zimbabwe) to assess the efficacy of the measles vaccine. The

---

* Correspondence: Tawanda Marufu, University of Zimbabwe College of Health Sciences, Box A 178, Avondale, Harare, Zimbabwe. E-mail: marufut@yahoo.com.

vaccine efficacy assessment was carried out on an epidemiological basis by relating measles transmission in the vaccinated and unvaccinated children aged 10-23 months. Measles cases were identified on the basis of a standard case definition and data on occurrence of measles cases was collected through an active surveillance system. Efficacies of 73%, 82% and 77% were calculated for the years 1987, 1988 and 1989 respectively. Over the three year period mean efficacy was found to be 77% (95% CI: 75-79%). The vaccine efficacies found in this study were lower than 85% which is the officially accepted efficacy of the measles vaccine that is in use in Zimbabwe. The low vaccine efficacy found in this study is attributed to the fact that the measles vaccine is applied (at nine months of age) when probably 10-20% of children still have prenatally acquired maternal antibodies. It is suggested that further studies be carried out in Zimbabwe to enable the country to determine the way forward.

INTRODUCTION

In Zimbabwe in recent years there has been concern over the rise in the number of measles cases among measles vaccinees (also called vaccine failures) and the role these cases are playing in maintaining measles transmission. Of the measles cases reported to the Ministry of Health, measles vaccination failures now outnumber unvaccinated cases and the number of vaccination failures is above what is expected in relation to the vaccine efficacy of 85% (85% is the officially accepted measles vaccine efficacy in Zimbabwe (1)). On account of this concern questions have been raised about the efficacy of the measles vaccine that is in use in Zimbabwe. This paper examines an assessment of the vaccine efficacy study which was carried out in Gweru as a result of similar concerns.

Gweru, the capital city of Midlands province in Zimbabwe, has a population of 140806 (1992 national population census). In Gweru, children were vaccinated against measles at 9 months of age with a Schwarz-type vaccine (0.5 mls or 1000 $TCID_{50}$). Vaccinations were carried out at static primary care health facilities on a “supermarket” approach basis. Vaccination coverage rose from 7% in 1971 (when vaccination against measles was commenced) to 90% in 1986. After 1985 the number of measles cases among measles vaccinees began to rise. Initially this was attributed to cold chain failure. The whole cold chain process was examined and efforts were made to ensure that the cold chain was functioning well. This entailed ensuring proper storage of vaccines with respect to recommended temperatures from the time vaccines are received to the time of use. Despite this effort, by 1986 the number of measles cases among measles vaccinees had outstripped the unvaccinated cases. On account of this the Public Health Department in Gweru decided to carry out a study to assess the efficacy of the measles vaccine. The study was carried out over a three year period, 1987 to 1989.

OUR STUDY

The study was prospective in nature. The assessment of the measles vaccine efficacy was carried out on an epidemiological basis by relating transmission of the disease among the vaccinated and unvaccinated children. Only children aged 10-23 months were included in the study. This was meant to exclude children who got the disease at or before nine months of age (who would not have been affected by the vaccination effort) and those aged 24 months or older (whose vaccinations had occurred in the past and therefore their involvement in the study would not relate to the efficacy of the vaccine that was in current use at the time). Only children who had measles vaccination at 9 months of age were included in the study. This was because the vaccine efficacy which was being assessed related to the official age of measles vaccination in Zimbabwe which is 9 months of age (2).

Measles cases were identified on the basis of a standard case definition which was availed to all primary health care facilities in the city, the city's infectious disease hospital and personnel who were assigned to investigate measles cases in the community. Age and vaccination status data on all measles cases reported from primary care facilities and the infectious disease hospital and those cases identified during case investigations in the community were entered on a special surveillance form. On this form an indication was made of the age of the person with the disease, vaccination status (whether vaccinated or not), age at vaccination (including the facility where the person was vaccinated), date of vaccination (where applicable), date of commencement of the disease and its signs and symptoms (in relation to the standard case definition of the disease).

Data on measles vaccinations (at 9 months of age) was collected monthly from all the city's primary health care institutions. At the end of every year the vaccination coverage was calculated by relating total measles vaccinations for the year to the population which was eligible for vaccination as per population census figures.

The measles vaccine efficacy was assessed annually by use of the formula developed by Orenstein et al. (3):

$$VE = \frac{\text{AR in unvaccinated} - \text{AR in vaccinated}}{\text{AR unvaccinated}} \times 100$$

where AR is the attack rate and VE is the vaccine efficacy

An estimate of the expected number of vaccinated children who would get the disease (vaccine failures) if the vaccine efficacy were 85% was made from this study. This was done by use of the formula developed by Orenstein et al. (3):

$$PVC = \frac{PPV - (PPV \times VE)}{1 - (PPV \times VE)}$$

where PCV is the percentage of vaccinated cases, PPV is the percentage of population vaccinated (vaccination coverage) and VE is the vaccine efficacy.

The study had the following limitations: (1) There were problems with the definition of vaccination status of cases particularly where there was no documentary proof. Seven such cases occurred in 1987 and two in 1988, giving 1.3% of all measles cases reported for the period 1987 to 1989. It was therefore decided that in the absence of documentary proof (child health card) such a case of measles would be deemed unvaccinated; (2) An effort was made to investigate cases in the community to avoid missing unreported cases (including deaths). There is no doubt that this effort was met with some success, but it is equally possible that some cases could have been missed in investigations; and (3) Elsewhere efficacy studies of this nature have often been carried out during measles epidemics. This has its obvious advantages. Efficacy studies carried out in relation to an epidemiological entity or occurrence like an epidemic take a much shorter time to carry out. Completeness in identifying all cases involved is probably easier (as opposed to being on the lookout for sporadic cases) and denominators to be used in calculating attack rates relate to populations which are affected by the epidemic only. Unfortunately such an opportunity did not avail itself during the three years of the study.

FINDINGS

In the age group 10-23 months some 53, 39 and 18 measles cases were reported for the years 1987, 1988 and 1989 respectively. Measles vaccination failures among measles cases aged 10-23 months contributed 73.6%, 64.1% and 77.8% in the years 1987, 1988 and 1989 respectively. If the measles vaccine efficacy were 85% (as officially accepted in Zimbabwe) vaccine failures among children aged 10-23 months would have accounted for 52%, 63% and 60% among reported measles in the years 1987, 1988 and 1989 respectively. Calculations of measles vaccine efficacy found efficacies of 73%, 82% and 77% for the years 1987, 1988 and 1989 respectively. Over the three year study period mean efficacy was found to be 77% (95% CI: 75-79%) (see tables 1 and 2).

Table1. Age and vaccination status of measles cases reported in the city of Gweru, 1987-89

	Age group (Months)							
	0-9	**10-23**		**24-119**		**120+**		
Year		**+**	**-**	**+**	**-**	**+**	**-**	**Reported cases**
1987	20	39	14	142	31	7	14	267
1988	19	25	14	133	63	3	14	271
1989	19	14	4	71	35	1	20	164

+Vaccinated.
-Unvaccinated.

Table2. Measles vaccination coverage, Percentage of vaccinated cases, Expected percentage of vaccinated cases if vaccine efficacy were 85%, Incidence rates in the vaccinated and unvaccinated and vaccine efficacies for the years 1987- 1989 for the child population aged 10-23 months in the City of Gweru

	1987	1988	1989
Vaccination coverage (PPV)	88 %	92 %	91%
PCV	73%	64%	77%
Expected PCV if VE were 85%	52%	63%	60%
Incidence rates in the vaccinated per 100 000 population	945	1 041	330
Incidence rates in the unvaccinated per 100 000 population	3 500	5 785	1 420
Vaccine efficacy	73%	82%	77%

VE: vaccine efficacy. PPV: % of population vaccinated (vaccine coverage).
PCV: % of cases vaccinated (Vaccine failures).

Discussion

An increase in the proportion of cases which occur among children previously vaccinated (vaccine failures) is ordinarily an expected outcome of high vaccination coverage and does not signify failure of the vaccination program (4-6). However, the increase in the number of vaccine failures as found in this study assumes significance in that the proportion of vaccine failures is more than what would be expected if the measles vaccine efficacy were 85%. This is an indication that the vaccine efficacy is probably lower than 85%.

In this study vaccine efficacies of 73%, 81% and 77% were found in Gweru. In a measles vaccine efficacy assessment study carried out during a measles epidemic in the City of Harare (Zimbabwe) in 1988 an efficacy of 73% was found for children aged 9-24 months in the absence of evidence of cold chain failure (7).

Findings of low vaccine efficacy in the Gweru study could be attributed to many factors, the commonest of which are cold chain failure and the effect of prenatally acquired maternal antibodies (2,7-11). In the current study, as in Harare city, efforts were put into ensuring that the cold chain was functioning well during the entire study period. Also, account has to be taken of the fact that the measles vaccine which is now in use is a lot more heat stable than the vaccine which was in use at the inception of measles vaccination in the late 1960s (8). Outbreak investigations in developing countries have documented vaccine efficacy rates of 70-90%. These studies include Point Noire (VE = 78%), Congo (VE = 87%). Tanzania (VE = 96%) and a recent study in rural Burundi (VE = 72%). In these studies it has been observed that even under good cold chain conditions, measles vaccine efficacy in developing is lower than in industrialized countries because the vaccine is applied when 10-20% of children still have transplacentally acquired maternal antibodies (11).

In recent years there have been reports to the effect that there is impaired humoral response to measles vaccine in HIV infected children (12). With the HIV epidemic on the increase in the 1990s in most developing countries there is therefore the possibility that there may be an increase in vaccination failures on account of this. However, in this study the observed vaccination failures could not be attributed to the effect of HIV infection in children because the study was carried out before the HIV epidemic had taken root in Zimbabwe (13).

In conclusion, the efficacy of the vaccine that is in use in Zimbabwe is probably lower than the 85%. This would explain why the proportion of vaccinated cases (vaccine failures) is higher than what would be expected if the vaccine efficacy were 85%. If the vaccine efficacy is as low as was found in this study it means that on a single dose measles vaccination regime high vaccination coverage (of over 90%) would need to be maintained over a long period of time in order for measles morbidity rates to decline. It also means that it would be difficult to break measles transmission cycles because measles vaccination failures would be part of the pool of susceptibles and would therefore ensure continued transmission of the disease. There is an urgent need for more vaccine efficacy studies to be carried out in Zimbabwe to enable the country to define the way forward. These studies should include an examination of the cold chain and its effect on the potency of the vaccines at various points of use and the effect of transplacentally acquired maternal antibodies on the efficacy of the measles vaccine.

ACKNOWLEDGMENTS

This chapter is a revised version of an original paper published in the Central African Journal of Medicine (Marufu T, Siziya S, Manyame B, Xaba E, Silape Z, Zimbizi P, Ruwodo C, Mason E, Matchaba-Hove R, Mudyarabikwa O. Questioning the level of efficacy of the measles vaccine in use in Zimbabwe. Central African Journal of Medicine 1995; 41: 241-5) and the authors have obtained the permission from Central African Journal of Medicine to use this material.

REFERENCES

[1] MOHCW. Weekly report on rapid notification of diseases, deaths and health events: Public Health Surveillance Unit – Ministry of Health and Child Welfare (Zimbabwe). Week no. 40 ending 9 October 1994;3:5-13.

[2] ZEPI. Zimbabwe Expanded Programme on Immunization: plan of operations (1986-90). Harare: Government of the Republic of Zimbabwe, 1986: 4.

[3] Orenstein WA, Bernier RH, Dondero TJ, Hinman AR, Marks JS, Bart KJ, Sirotkin B. Field evaluation of vaccine efficacy. Bull World Health Organ 1985;63:1055-68.

[4] EPI. Global Advisory Group on Expanded Programme on Immunization 12th meeting, 16-20 October 1989 Tokyo, Japan.

[5] Marufu T. The changing age of ecology of measles and its implications on measles control. Cent Afr J Med 1992; 38: 208-14.

[6] Cutts F. Measles control in the 1990s: Principles for the next Decade. Geneva: WHO/EPI/GEN/90.2, 1990:14.

[7] Kambarami RA, Nathoo KJ, Nkrumah FK, Pirie DJ. Measles epidemic in Harare, Zimbabwe despite high measles immunization coverage rates. Bull World Health Organ 1991; 69:213-9.

[8] Editorial. Rationalizing measles vaccination. Lancet 1981; II: 236-7.

[9] Cutts F. Measles- the immunological basis for immunization. Geneva: WHO/EPI/GEN/93.17, 1993: 6-10.

[10] Nizar A. Vaccination. Lyon: Institut Merieux, 1986:14-5.

[11] Foster S, McFarland DA. Measles: Health sector priorities review. Atlanta, GA: World Bank/CDC, 1991:10 -11.

[12] AI-Attar I, Reisman J, Muehlmann M, McIntosh K. Decline of measles antibody titres after immunization in human immunodeficiency virus infected children. Pediatr Infect Dis J 1995; 14:149-51.

[13] Bassett MT, Latif AS, Katzenstein DA, Emmanuel JC. Sexual behaviour and risk factors for HIV infection in a group of male factory workers who donated blood in Harare, Zimbabwe. J Acquired Immune Defic Syndr 1992; 5:556-9.

SECTION TWO: USE OF MULTIPLE DOSE MEASLES VACCINATION STRATEGIES IN THE CONTROL OF MEASLES

In: Measles
Editors: T. Marufu, S. Siziya et al.

ISBN: 978-1-63485-559-4

Chapter 6

IMPACT OF MULTIPLE DOSE MEASLES VACCINATION ON MEASLES TRANSMISSION PATTERNS

Tawanda Marufu*, MBChB, MSc and Seter Siziya, BA (Ed), MSc, PhD
Department of Community Medicine,
University of Zimbabwe Medical School, Avondale,
Harare, Zimbabwe

Multiple dose measles vaccination was applied in Gweru, Zimbabwe in 1990-1996. This included (a) a vaccine administered to children at 9 months of age and revaccination of the same children at any point between ages 12 and 23 months, and (b) a single mass vaccination campaign targeted at children aged 12-119 months (who were vaccinated irrespective of vaccination status or disease history) run in early 1990. This study describes the impact of this schedule on measles transmission patterns. Using measles surveillance data the study compared measles transmission patterns under single dose vaccination in 1983-1989 and under multiple dose vaccination in 1990-1996. Median measles incidence rates were 261.0 and 19.0/100 000 population in 1983-89 and 1990-1996, respectively, and these rates were different ($p = 0.002$). Vaccinated cases (vaccine failures) among children aged 10-119 months significantly

* Correspondence: Tawanda Marufu, University of Zimbabwe College of Health Sciences, Box A 178, Avondale, Harare, Zimbabwe. E-mail: marufut@yahoo.com.

increased from 49.6 to 70.4% of all reported measles cases in 1983-1989 and had a median incidence rate of 480.4/100 000. In 1990-1996 the median incidence rate was 12.8 and these incidence rates were different (p = 0.002).Cases aged 60-119 months significantly increased from 14.3 to 62.2% of all reported measles cases in 183-1989 and had a median incidence rate of 654.1/100 000. In 1990-1996 the median incidence rate was 21.4 and these incidence rates were different (p = 0.004). It was concluded that under multiple dose vaccination regime, lower measles incidence rates occurred most likely due to reduction in both vaccine failures and cases aged 60-119 moths.

INTRODUCTION

The city of Gweru in Zimbabwe has a population of 124,735. Measles vaccination was commenced in 1971 in Gweru. In 1971-89 a single dose of live hyperattenuated Schwarz strain vaccine (0.5 mls or 1,000 $TCID_{50}$) was administered to children at 9 months of age at the city's static health facilities. At vaccine coverage rates of >80% in 1985-89 measles incidence rates were declining (1). In this period it was observed that among reported measles cases, vaccinated cases (vaccine failures) and cases aged >60 months, most of whom had had vaccination, were increasing (2, 3). By 1989 there was concern that a buildup of susceptibles, in the form of vaccine failures or cases aged >60 months who were outside the primary target age group of the Expanded Programme of Immunization, could lead to epidemics in the future. It was decided that multiple dose vaccination strategy be employed to change these new transmission patterns. A project that implemented this strategy was run in Gweru in 1990-1996. In this chapter we report on changes in measles transmission patterns which occurred after this intervention.

OUR STUDY

Administration of multiple dose vaccination among children in Gweru was run as a quasi-experimental community intervention with both internal and external comparisons. This study, an internal comparison, compared occurrence of measles in the pre- and post-intervention periods. The hypothesis of this study was: at high coverage rates for vaccine that is applied at 9 months of age the incidence rates of measles would decline. Despite this decline, however, there would be an increase in occurrence of vaccine failures and cases aged >60 months with the potential of these susceptibles accumulating and causing epidemics in the future. Multiple dose measles vaccination strategy could reduce occurrence of these susceptibles thus averting the occurrence of epidemics and maintaining low measles transmission.

A two-pronged strategy was used in the provision of multiple doses of measles vaccine. The first variant of this strategy was that of a rapid and comprehensive "clean up" vaccination campaign targeted at all children aged 10-119 months (regardless of disease history or vaccination status) to clear this population of susceptibles. This campaign was carried in over a two weeks period in early 1990. In the second variant of the strategy, children that had had vaccination at 9 months of age at the city's static health facilities were given another single dose (revaccination) at any point between ages of 12 months and 23 months at the same facilities. This second strategy was implemented over the rest of the project period from immediately after the mass vaccination campaign of early 1990.

In Gweru, routine vaccinations are indicated on child health cards, and vaccination figures are compiled monthly. From 1990 revaccinations were also indicated on child health cards and revaccination figures were also compiled monthly. Vaccinations applied during the mass vaccine campaign of 1990 were indicated on child health cards. Children that did not have child health cards had new ones issued to them on which the campaign vaccination was indicated. Records or figures that were compiled after the campaign indicated the number of children vaccinated in the various age groups 12-23, 24-59 and 60-119 months.

Gweru has had active measles surveillance since 1967. Measles cases are identified on the basis of a standard clinical case definition that is available to staff at all health facilities. There are personnel who are assigned to investigate occurrence of unreported infectious diseases (including measles cases) within communities (active case search). Measles surveillance /investigation forms that have been in use indicate age at infection, gender, presenting features of the disease, need for hospitalization or not, treatment regime applied, outcome of illness (alive or dead), and occurrence of any other cases in relation to the identified case (which would also be investigated). Indication of vaccination status of cases was added to the surveillance form in January 1980. When the multiple-dose vaccination project was commenced in 1990 a slot was added to the surveillance form to indicate whether a case had had vaccination during the campaign of 1990 or routine revaccination, or none of the above. Information from measles surveillance forms was compiled monthly.

Measles vaccination and disease surveillance data for the period before and after intervention were analyzed. The study compared: (a) Vaccine coverage rates for the vaccine applied at 9 months of age in 1983-1989 and 1990-1996 (b) Occurrence of measles in 1983-89 and during the project period, 1990-1996. The following analyses were carried out:

a) Student's t-test was used to compare means of normally distributed data.
b) The Kruskal – Wallis test was used to compare medians of non-normally distributed data.
c) The linear trend was determined using chi-squared for linear trend.
d) The cut-off point for statistical significance was 5%.

The main outcome measures were:

a) Measles vaccine coverage rates for the vaccine applied at 9 months of age in 1983-1989 and 1990-1996.
b) Vaccine coverage rates in various age groups for the vaccine applied during the 1990 measles mass vaccination campaign and vaccine coverage rates for the revaccination applied at 12-23 months of age in 1990-1996.
c) Measles incidence rates in Gweru city in 1983-1989 and 1990-1996.
d) Measles incidence rate among vaccinated children aged 10-119 months in 1983-1989 and 1990-1996
e) Measles incidence rates in children aged 60-119 months in 1983-1989 and 1990-1996.

FINDINGS

In 1983-1989 and 1990-1996 vaccine coverage rates for the measles vaccine applied at 9 months of age were 72.0-92.0% (mean = 84.6, SD = 7.7) and 87.0-92.0% (mean = 89.7, SD = 1.7), respectively. In the two periods the vaccine coverage rates were not significantly different (p = 0.109). Coverage rates for the revaccination of children at 12-23 months of age in 1990-1996 were 81.0-87.0% (mean = 82.4, SD = 2.1). Vaccine coverage rates for 1990 mass campaign were 83.0, 87.0 and 89.0% in children aged 12-23, 24-59 and 60-119 months, respectively.

In 1983-1989 measles incidence rates in Gweru were 151.0-450.0/100,000 population (median = 261.0, Q_1 = 156.0, Q_3 = 400.0) while in 1990-1996 these incidence rate were 9-29/100 000 population (median = 19.0, Q_1 = 13.0, Q_3 = 22.0). In the two period the incidence rates were significantly different (p = 0.002). In 1983-1989 measles incidence rate declined linearly (X^2 for linear trend = 88.83, p<0.001) as shown in Figure 1.

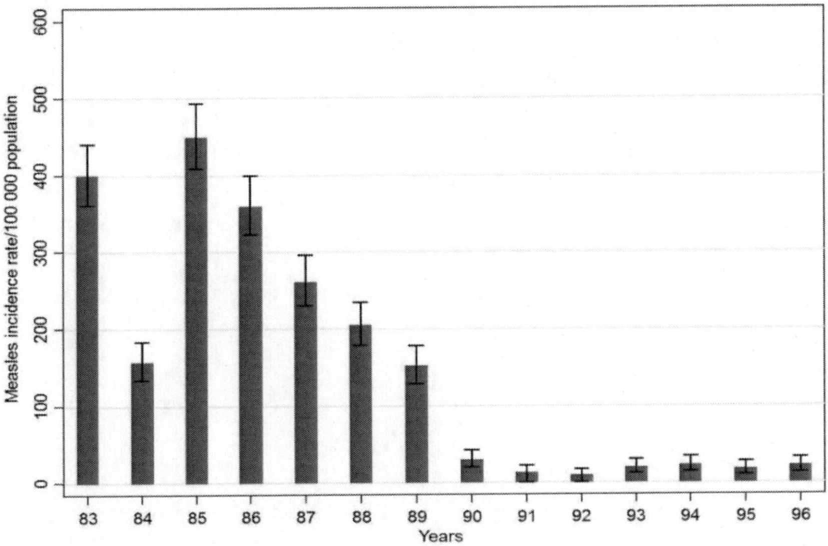

Figure1. Measles incidence rates in the city of Gweru in 1983-1996.

In 1983-1989 cases aged 10-119 months accounted for 97.5-99.3% (mean = 98.0, SD = 0.71) of all reported measles cases in Gweru. In this period 26-248 vaccinated measles cases (median = 188.0, Q_1 = 86.0, Q_3 = 208.0) were identified. Vaccinated cases (vaccine failures) accounted for 49.6-70.4% (median = 53.1, Q_1 = 47.1, Q_3 = 59.4) of reported cases in this age group and the proportion of vaccine failures significantly increased in this period (X^2 fore linear trend = 4.367, p = 0.037). Incidence rates of vaccine failures in this age group during this period were 77.7-701.5/100 000 (median = 480.4, Q_1 = 200.3, Q_3 = 621.0). In 1990-1996 all 11-35 measles cases (median = 24.0, Q_1 = 16.0, Q_3 = 30) that were reported in Gweru were aged 10-119 months. Of these 4-15 cases (median = 9.0, Q_1 = 5.0, Q_3 = 11.0) had had vaccination. Incidence rates of vaccinated measles cases in this age group in this period were 7.3-33.5/100 000 (median = 12.8, Q_1 = 8.2, Q_3 = 21.8).

Incidence of vaccinated measles cases in age group 10-119 months in 1983-1989 and 1990-1996 were significantly different ($p = 0.002$).

During 1983-1989 some 7-173 cases (median = 128.0, Q_1 = 89.0, Q_3 = 147.0) aged 60-119 months were reported. Cases in this age group accounted for 14.3-62.2% (median = 37.6, Q_1 = 22.0, Q_3 = 54.2) of all reported cases and among all reported cases the proportion of cases in this age group significantly increased in this period (X^2 for linear trend = 82.059, $p < 0.001$). Some 49.0-82.0% of cases (median = 62.0, Q_1 = 50.0, Q_3 = 68.0) reported in this age group during this period were vaccine failure. Incidence rates of measles in age group 60-119 months in 1983-1989 were 41.9-978.9/100 000 (median = 654.1, Q_1 = 414.6, Q_3 = 719.6). In 1990-1996 among all reported measles cases 5-21 cases (median = 10.0, Q_1 = 5.0, Q_3 = 21.0) were aged 60-119 months. Of these 1-7 (median = 3.0, Q_1 = 1.0, Q_3 = 7.0) had had measles vaccination. Incidence rates of measles in this age group in this period were 7.3-93.7/100 000 (median = 21.4, Q_1 = 14.2, Q_3 = 49.5). Incidence rates in age group 60-119 months in 1983-1989 and 1990-1996 were significantly different ($p = 0.004$).

DISCUSSION

The current study has shown that although measles incidence rates declined in 1983-1989 they were higher in that period compared 1990-1996. The higher level of occurrence of measles in 1983-89 (when compared to 1990-1996) could mostly be attributed to higher rates of occurrence of cases aged 60-119 months and higher rates of occurrence of vaccine failures among children aged 10-119 months.

Occurrence of vaccine failures is blamed on a vaccine of less than 100% efficacy (2, 4, 5) or waning immunity in immunized persons (2, 4, 6). As was experienced in Gweru in 1983-1989, at high vaccination coverage rates for vaccine applied at 9 months of age most measles transmission was sustained by vaccine failures (4, 5, 7). Accumulation of vaccine failures in developing countries or areas with moderate to high vaccine coverage rate has led to epidemics after a decline in measles transmission (4, 6). In 1990-1996 occurrence of vaccine failures in Gweru would have been minimized, thus reducing the potential for epidemics, on account of either the mass vaccination campaign of 1990, which led to revaccination of person who had had vaccination prior to the campaign, or routine revaccination applied to children at 12-23 months of age, which occurred over the rest of the project period.

Revaccination is known to improve vaccine efficacy thereby reducing occurrence of vaccine failures (8-10).

High rates of measles among children aged 60 months or older observed in Gweru in 1983-89 (compared to 1990-1996) have occurred in some developing countries or areas with high vaccine coverage rates similar to those of Gweru (4, 6, 11). As in Gweru, this occurrence has involved both vaccinated and unvaccinated cases (6, 11). The explanation for this has been that for vaccine applied in infancy, vaccination of a large proportion of the community reduces chances of susceptibles being exposed to the infectious agent in infancy, such that they would be exposed at an older age leading to an increase in average age at infection (4). High occurrences of cases in older children aged 60 months or older has been attended with epidemics (4, 7). In Gweru in 1990-1996 rates of cases in the age group 60-119 months were lower than in 1983-1989. It is likely that the mass measles vaccination campaign of 1990, that had high coverage rates in this age group, reduced occurrence of cases through either revaccination or reaching unvaccinated individuals that had missed vaccination at 9 months of age. There is therefore a distinct possibility that this campaign may have reduced the epidemic potential in this age group in 1990-1996 thus averting occurrence of epidemics as has been observed elsewhere.

Vaccine coverage rates for the vaccine applied at 9 months of age were as high in 1990-1996 as they were in 1983-1989 and this may have minimized occurrence of unvaccinated measles cases in both periods. However, the lower incidence rates of measles observed in Gweru in 1990-1996 (compared to the earlier period) could partially be explained by the effect of the vaccination campaign of 1990 that reached unvaccinated susceptibles in the various age groups that were included in the campaign.

In conclusion, high measles vaccine coverage rates of >80% of single dose vaccine applied at 9 months of age in 1983-1989 led to a decline in measles incidence rates. Application of multiple dose measles vaccination of coverage rates of >80% in 1990-1996 led to lower incidence rates compared to earlier period. Multiple dose measles vaccination may have reduced incidence rates of both vaccine failure among children aged 10-119 months and cases among children aged 60-119 months to achieve overall reduction in measles incidence rates in 1990-1996 compared to the earlier period.

Acknowledgments

This chapter is a revised version of an original paper published in the Journal of Tropical Pediatrics (Marufu T, Siziya S. Impact of Multiple dose measles vaccination on measles transmission patterns. Journal of Tropical Pediatrics 2001; 47: 335-8) and the authors have obtained the permission from Journal of Tropical Pediatrics to use this material.

References

[1] Marufu T. The changing age ecology of measles and its implications on measles control. Cent Afr J Med 1992; 38:208-14.

[2] Marufu T, Siziya S, Manyame B, Xaba E, Silape-Marufu Z, Zimbizi P, et al. Questioning the level of efficacy of the measles vaccine in use in Zimbabwe. Cent Afr J Med 1995; 41: 241-5.

[3] Marufu T, Murugasampillary S, Siziya S, Manyame B, Silape-Marufu Z, Xaba E, et al. Is the protection afforded measles vaccinees the same in children of all age groups? Is the protection afforded measles vaccinees the same in children of all age groups? Cent Afr J Med 1995; 41: 144-7.

[4] Global Programme for Vaccines and Immunization. Immunization policy. Expanded programme on immunization. Geneva: WHO/EPI/GEN 95.3, 1995.

[5] Expanded Programme on Immunization. Global measles strategy picks up pace. EPI Newsletter 1994; XVI: 3.

[6] Coetzee N, Hussey GD, Visser G, Baron P, Keen A. The 1992 measles epidemic in Cape Town: A changing epidemiological pattern. S Afr Med J 1994; 84: 145-9.

[7] Expanded Programme on Immunization. Measles control in the 1990s: plan of action for measles control 1992. Geneva: WHO/EPI/GEN/92.3, 1992.

[8] Marufu T, Siziya S, Tshimanga M, Murugasampillay S, Mason E. Comparison of protection afforded by single measles vaccination and late revaccination schedules. E Afr Med J 1997; 74: 777-9.

[9] Rosenthal SR, Clemens CJ. Two-dose measles vaccination schedules. Bull World Health Organ 1993; 71: 421-8.

[10] Global Programme for Vaccines. Measles control in the 1990s: Final draft report of the GPV/CVI informal consultation on strategies to accelerate global measles control. Washington DC: EPI/WHO, 1994.

[11] Khuri-Bhulos NA. Measles in Jordan: A prototype of the problems with measles in developing countries. Pediatr Infect Dis J 1995; 14: 22-6.

In: Measles
Editors: T. Marufu, S. Siziya et al.
ISBN: 978-1-63485-559-4

Chapter 7

COMPARISON OF PROTECTION AFFORDED BY SINGLE MEASLES VACCINATION AND LATE REVACCINATION SCHEDULES

Tawanda Marufu[1,*], MB ChB, MSc,
Seter Siziya[1], BA (Ed), MSc, PhD,
Mufuta Tshimanga[1], MD, MPH,
Shiva Murugasampillay[2], MBBS, MSc
and Elizabeth Mason[2], MBChB, MSc
[1]Department of Community Medicine,
University of Zimbabwe Medical School, Harare, Zimbabwe
[2]WHO Country Office, Harare, Zimbabwe

An intervention study compared the protection afforded vaccines by single measles vaccination and late revaccination schedules in 1990-94. During the intervention a single revaccination (after initial vaccination at nine months of age) was applied to children at any point in time between 12 and 23 months of age. Cases of measles aged 10-23 months were identified through an active surveillance system and in this period 5, 11 and 11 cases of revaccinated, single vaccination and unvaccinated children were identified. Measles incidence rates were 392.2-415.6 (mean = 405.6, SD = 6.7), 75.4-112.1 (mean = 91.7, SD = 13.3) and 12.8-

---

* Correspondence: Tawanda Marufu, University of Zimbabwe College of Health Sciences, Box A 178, Avondale, Harare, Zimbabwe. E-mail: marufut@yahoo.com.

15.2 (mean = 13.9, SD = 0.99) per 100 000 population in children who were unvaccinated, with single vaccination and revaccinated respectively. Relative risk of contracting measles in children who were unvaccinated or with single vaccination was 26.5-32.5 (mean = 29.4, SD = 2.3) and 5.8-8.8 (mean = 6.8, SD = 1.2) respectively compared with revaccinated children. Vaccine efficacies that were determined were 73 -81% (mean = 77.2, SD = 2.9) and 96.2-96.9% (mean = 96.6, SD = 0.27) for single vaccination schedules respectively. It was concluded that late revaccination affords vaccinees better protection than single vaccination through improvement in vaccine efficacy.

INTRODUCTION

Gweru, third largest city in Zimbabwe, has a population of 124,735 (1992 census). In Gweru, measles vaccination was commenced in 1971. A single dose of live hyper attenuated Schwarz strain vaccine (0.5 mls or 1,000 $TCID_{50}$) is applied to children at 9 months of age at the city's static health facilities. At vaccination coverage of 88 -91% in 1987-89 it was observed that the proportion of cases who were vaccinated among children aged 10-23 months was more than the expected if the measles vaccine efficacy were 85%, the official efficacy of the measles vaccine that is currently in use in Zimbabwe. Vaccine efficacy studies which were carried out over a three year period in Gweru found efficacies of 73-81% (95% CI: 75-79%) (1, 2). It was postulated that the low vaccine efficacy could have been occasioned by the effect of transplacentally acquired maternal antibodies which neutralized the vaccine when it is applied at 9 months of age. It was therefore hypothesized that revaccination of these children (at an age when it was assumed that maternal antibodies would have totally decayed) would afford vaccinees better protection through improvement of vaccine efficacy. On the basis of this hypothesis a project was carried out to determine the efficacy of measles revaccination schedules for the period 1990-1994. The study compared protection afforded vaccinees by single vaccination and revaccination schedules. In the city of Gweru urban district measles revaccination project was run over a seven years, 1990- 1996. The determination of efficacy of measles revaccination which was carried out over the four year period 1990-94 was one of the specific objectives of the measles revaccination project of 1990-96.

OUR STUDY

A two-pronged strategy was employed in the provision of late measles revaccination. The first variant of this strategy was that of a rapid and comprehensive "clean up" vaccination campaign targeted at all children aged 12 months to 10 years to clear this population of all susceptibles. This campaign was carried out over a two week period in early 1990. In the second strategy children who had had measles vaccination at 9 months of age at the city's static health facilities were provided another single dose (revaccination) at any point in time between the ages of 12 and 23 months at the same facilities. This second strategy was employed over the rest of the project period 1991-1996.

Both the initial vaccination (at 9 months of age) and the revaccination were indicated on the children's child health cards. Records of initial vaccination at 9 months of age and revaccination were compiled monthly. A cross-sectional survey was carried out in the community in 1993 to determine vaccination coverage for both initial vaccination at 9 months of age and the revaccination in children aged 12 -23 months.

The city of Gweru has an active measles surveillance system. In this system cases are identified on the basis of a standard case definition which is available to staff at all primary health care facilities and the city's infectious disease hospital. There are personnel who are assigned to investigate occurrence of unreported infectious diseases (including measles cases) within communities (active case search). Measles surveillance investigation forms which have been in use indicate age at infection, vaccination status, gender, presenting features of disease, need for hospitalization or lack of it, treatment regime and occurrence of any other cases in relation to an identified case (which would also be investigated). On this form a slot was added which would indicate whether the case had revaccination or not. Data from the measles surveillance system were compiled monthly.

Every year, the Town Clerk's office in the city of Gweru carries out census surveys that determine the population for which various services would be provided. Information from these census surveys was used on this project to determine the vaccine requirements in relation to numbers of the eligible population and in the calculation of both vaccination coverage rates and measles incidence rates.

During the project, at the end of each calendar year vaccination coverage rates for initial vaccination at 9 months of age and late revaccination were determined by relating total vaccinations for the year to the population which was eligible for such vaccinations as per population census figures. The vaccination figures for 1993 came from the coverage survey indicated above. Measles incidence rates were determined annually on the basis of cases identified through the surveillance system with the population census figures used as denominators. In each year efficacies of both single vaccination and revaccination schedules were assessed epidemiologically by use of a formula developed by Orenstein et al. (3).

$$VE = \frac{\text{AR (in unvaccinated cases) - AR (in single vaccination or revaccinated cases)}}{\text{AR in unvaccinated}} \times 100$$

where AR is the attack rate (or incidence rate) and VE is the vaccine efficacy.

To measure the protection afforded vaccinees by single vaccination and revaccination schedules the following were determined annually: (a) Incidence rates of measles among children aged 10-23 months that were not vaccinated (unvaccinated), children with single vaccination and revaccinated children; (b) Relative risk of contracting measles among unvaccinated children or children with single vaccination compared to the revaccinated children; (c) Efficacy of single vaccination and revaccination schedules.

Limitations of the study included: (i) Efforts were put into investigation of cases in the community (active case searches) to avoid missing unreported cases (including deaths).This effort was met with some success but it is possible that some cases could have been missed particularly subclinical cases, and (ii) There were a few problems with definition of vaccination status of cases particularly where there was no documentary proof (for example, child health card). Throughout the project period this affected seven people. These people were deemed unvaccinated. Fortunately these were all not aged 10-23 months and therefore would not affect the results of this study.

FINDINGS

Vaccination coverages for the initial vaccination at 9 months of age and late revaccination were 88.6-91.8% and 81.2-87.2% respectively in the period 1990 – 1994.

In the period under review 5, 11 and 11 measles cases who were revaccinated, with single vaccination and unvaccinated respectively were reported in the age group 10-23 months. Table 1 shows measles incidence rates for the 10-23 months age group among the three vaccinations status groups by year.

Table 1. Measles incidence rates/100 000 population in the age group 10-23 months among unvaccinated cases, cases with single vaccination and the revaccinated cases (1990-1994)

Year	Unvaccinated	Single vaccination	Revaccinated
1990	403.2	88.7	15.2
1991	407.6	93.6	14.5
1992	397.2	75.4	13.1
1993	404.3	88.9	13.7
1994	415.6	112.1	12.8

Measles incidence rates were 397.2-415.6 (mean = 405.6, SD = 6.7), 75.4-112.1 (median = 91.7, SD = 13.3), and 12.8-15.2 (mean = 13.9, SD = 0.99) per 100 000 population in unvaccinated, single vaccination and revaccinated children respectively.

Relative risk of contracting measles in unvaccinated children and those with single vaccination was 26.5-32.5 (mean = 29.4, SD = 2.3) and 5.8-8.8 (mean = 6.8, SD = 1.2) respectively compared with the revaccinated children (see Table 2).

Table 2. Relative risk of contracting measles in the age group 10-23 months in unvaccinated children and children with single vaccination compared to revaccinated children in the same age group

Year	Unvaccinated	Single vaccination	Revaccinated
1990	26.5	5.8	1
1991	28.1	6.5	1
1992	30.3	5.8	1
1993	29.5	6.5	1
1994	32.5	8.8	1

Table 3 shows vaccine efficacies assessed for the single vaccination and revaccination schedules in the period 1990-1994. Efficacies were 73-81% (mean = 72.2, SD = 2.9) and 96.2-96.9% (mean = 96.6, SD = 0.27) for the single vaccination and revaccination schedules respectively.

Table 3. Vaccine efficacies for the single dose and revaccination schedules

Year	Single vaccination	Revaccination
1990	78.0%	96.2%
1991	77.0%	96.4%
1992	81.0%	96.7%
1993	77.0%	96.6%
1994	73.0%	96.9%

DISCUSSION

In 1981 WHO's Expanded Programme on Immunization (EPI) recommended that measles vaccine be provided to children at 9 months of age. This age was meant to be a compromise or balance between two factors, the earliest age at which high rates of seroconversion can be obtained, and the age group with the highest risk of infection. Vaccinating earlier than 9 months would reduce vaccine efficacy due to interference with prenatally acquired maternal antibodies while vaccinating later than 9 months was associated with a higher vaccine efficacy but resulted in many children getting infection before reaching age of vaccination (4, 5). This study has confirmed that by applying the vaccine after 12 months of age (through revaccination) the efficacy is much higher compared to that of the single vaccination applied at 9 months of age.

Studies of measles vaccine efficacy in developing countries have found efficacies of 70-90%. These studies have included Point Noire (78%), Congo (87%), Tanzania (96%) and Burundi (72%) (5).The wide variation in efficacies could be due to methodologies used in the various studies. Vaccine efficacy studies carried out in Zimbabwe have consistently shown that the efficacy of the measles vaccine that is currently in use in Zimbabwe is low. These studies have included Gweru city (1987-1989, 73-81%) (1), Harare City (1988, 73%) (6), and Masvingo district (1995, 78.3%) (7). Efficacies of measles vaccination applied at 9 months of age found in this study are consistent with those found in similar studies from Zimbabwe. These low efficacies support the observation that even under good cold chain conditions, vaccine efficacy in developing countries is lower than in industrialized countries because vaccine is applied at an age when 10-20% of children still have maternal antibodies but vaccination cannot be delayed because of early age of infection (5).

In developing countries or areas with moderate to high vaccination coverage, epidemics have occurred after periods of low transmission (8, 9). These countries or areas have included Harare in Zimbabwe (6, 9), Muyinga Health Sector in Burundi (9,10), Lesotho and Swaziland (8). Among the many reasons cited for this occurrence has been the accumulation of primary vaccination failures (occurrence of measles among the vaccinated) (9). The current study has shown that the incidence rates of measles among the revaccinated is lower than that of children with single vaccination and that the risk of contracting measles in children with single vaccination is 5.8-8.8 times that of the revaccinated. This would mean that the revaccinated are afforded better vaccinal protection compared to those with single vaccination. Thus developing countries or areas with high vaccination coverage (for the vaccine applied at 9 months of age) might need to fortify vaccinees through revaccination to reduce the occurrence of vaccination failures who would maintain transmission despite the high vaccination coverage. The importance of vaccination failures in sustaining measles transmission has recently been brought to the fore by WHO's target of reducing measles incidence rates by 90% (of pre-immunization levels) in 1995 and after. It has been observed that even a100% coverage with a vaccine of 80% efficacy leaves 20% of vaccine recipients susceptible to measles, permitting continued transmission in the community, and falling short of the 90% reduction goal (11, 12). It is concluded that a late measles revaccination schedule affords vaccinees better protection through a higher efficacy than single vaccination applied at 9 months of age.

ACKNOWLEDGMENTS

This chapter is a revised version of an original paper published in the East African Medical Journal (Marufu T, Siziya S, Tshimanga M, Murugasampillay S, Mason E. Comparison of protection afforded by single measles vaccination and late revaccination schedules. East African Medical Journal 1997; 74:777-9) and the authors have obtained the permission from East African Medical Journal to use this material.

References

[1] Marufu T, Siziya S, Manyame B, Xaba E, Silape Z, Zimbizi P, et al. Questioning the level of efficacy of the measles vaccine that is in use in Zimbabwe. Cent Afr J Med 1995; 41:241-5.

[2] Marufu T. The changing age ecology of measles and its implications on measles control. Cent Afr J Med 1992; 38:208 -14.

[3] Orenstein WA, Bernier RH, Dondero TJ, Hinman AR, Marks JS, Bart KJ, et al. Field evaluation of vaccine efficacy. Bull World Health Organ 1985; 63:1055-68.

[4] Rosenthal SR, Clements CJ. Two-dose measles vaccination schedules. Bull World Health Organ 1993; 71:421-8.

[5] Foster SO, McFarland DA, John AM. Measles. In: Jamison DT, Mosley WH, Measham AR, Bobadilla JL, eds. Disease control priorities in developing countries. New York: Oxford University Press, 1993:161–87.

[6] Kambarami RA, Nathoo KJ, Nkrumah FK, Pirie DJ. Measles epidemic in Harare, Zimbabwe despite high measles immunization coverage rates. Bull World Health Organ 1991; 69:213-9.

[7] Mudzamiri WS, Peterson DE, Marufu T, Biellick R.J and L'Herminez M. Measles vaccine efficacy in Masvingo district, Zimbabwe. Cent Afr J Med 1996; 42:195-7.

[8] Cutts F. Measles control in the 1990's: Principles for the next decade. Expanded programme on immunization: Geneva: WHO/EPI/GEN/90.2, 1990.

[9] Global Programme for Vaccines and Immunization. Immunization policy. Expanded programme on immunization. Geneva: WHO/EPI/GEN/95.3, 1995.

[10] Chen TR, Weierbach R, Bissoffi Z, Cutts. F, Rhodes P, Ramaroso S, et al. 'Post honeymoon period' measles outbreak in Muyinga sector, Burundi. Int J Epidemiol 1994; 23:185-93.

[11] Expanded Programme on Immunization. Global measles strategy picks up pace. EPI Newsletter 1994:16:3.

[12] Global Programme for Vaccines. Measles Control in the 1990s: Final draft report of the GPV/CVI informal consultation on strategies to accelerate global measles control. Washington, DC: EPI/WHO, 1994.

In: Measles
Editors: T. Marufu, S. Siziya et al.

ISBN: 978-1-63485-559-4

Chapter 8

COMPARISON OF IMPACT OF SINGLE DOSE AND MULTIPLE DOSE MEASLES VACCINATION STRATEGIES ON MEASLES TRANSMISSION PATTERNS

Tawanda Marufu[1,*], MB ChB, MSc, Seter Siziya[2], BA (Ed), MSc, PhD and Willard Tinago[1], BSc, MSc, PhD

[1]Department of Community Medicine, College of Health Sciences, University of Zimbabwe, Harare, Zimbabwe

[2]Department of Clinical Sciences, Copperbelt University School of Medicine, Ndola, Zambia

Multiple dose measles vaccination intervention was applied in Gweru City, Zimbabwe, in 1990-96, following a single dose applied at 9 months of age during 1983-89. In the same periods in Bulawayo, only a single dose of measles vaccine was applied to children at 9 months of age. This study investigated the impact on measles transmission patterns of multiple dose measles vaccination strategy. Study design: Quasi-experimental community intervention applied in Gweru city with Bulawayo city as a control. The intervention included a single mass vaccination campaign carried out in1990 targeted at children aged 12-119

* Correspondence: Tawanda Marufu, University of Zimbabwe College of Health Sciences, Box A 178, Avondale, Harare, Zimbabwe. E-mail: marufut@yahoo.com.

months irrespective of their vaccination status or disease history. Children born after 1990 were vaccinated at 9 months of age plus another single dose applied at any point between ages of 12 and 23 months (revaccination). Measles cases were identified in both cities through surveillance. Mean coverage rates for measles vaccine applied at 9 months of age were in 1983-89 85.7% and 84.6% in Bulawayo and Gweru respectively, while in 1990-96 they were 89.0% and 89.7%, respectively. In both periods the vaccine coverage rates were not significantly different in the two cities (p = 0.464). In the 12-23 months age group, Gweru measles vaccination coverage rate in 1990 was 83% for single dose and 82.4% for second dose in 1990-96. Measles incidence rates in 1983-89 in both cities significantly declined and were not significantly different (p = 0.898). Median incidence rates of measles in1990-96 were 131.0 and 19.0/100,000 population in Bulawayo and Gweru respectively and these were significantly different (p = 0.021). Bulawayo had measles epidemics in 1992, 1993, 1994 and 1996. In Bulawayo in 1993-96 vaccinated measles cases accounted for a median of 58% of all reported cases aged 10-119 months. Median incidence rates of measles among vaccine failures aged 10-119 months in 1993-96 in Bulawayo and Gweru were 419.1 and 13.1/100 000 population respectively and these incidence rates were significantly different (p = 0.021). In Bulawayo in 1993-96 cases aged 60-119 months accounted for a median of 56.5% of all reported cases. Median incidence rates of measles among cases aged 60-119 months in 1993-96 in Bulawayo and Gweru were 869.9 and 26.9/100 000 population respectively and these rates were significantly different (p = 0.021). Conclusion: Multiple dose vaccination strategies led to significantly reduced measles transmission in Gweru (compared to Bulawayo) in 1990-1996 by minimizing occurrence of vaccine failures and occurrence of cases in older children aged 60-119 months.

INTRODUCTION

A study was carried out to determine the impact of single dose and multiple dose measles vaccination strategies on occurrence of measles. The study compared occurrence of measles in Gweru (population: 124,735) and Bulawayo (population: 620 936) cities in Zimbabwe in1983-89 when both cities had a strategy that solely entailed applying measles vaccine at nine months of age and in1990-96 when multiple dose vaccination strategies were applied in Gweru while.

Bulawayo continued to apply measles vaccination to children aged 9 months.

OUR STUDY

Application of multiple dose measles vaccination strategy among children in the city of Gweru was a quasi-experimental community intervention with both internal and external comparisons:

(a) Internal comparison or "self-controlled" intervention (before and after) aspect of the study in Gweru has already been described (1) and (b) External comparison or external "control." The purpose of this chapter is to describe this aspect of the study by comparing measles transmission patterns in Gweru where the intervention was carried and Bulawayo, the "control", where the intervention was not carried out.

The hypothesis of the study was that: At high coverage rates of measles vaccine applied to children at nine months of age measles incidence rates would decline. Despite this decline, however, there would be an increase in occurrence of vaccine failures (occurrence of cases among vaccinated children) and a shift of disease to a school-going children population aged 60-110 months. High occurrence of vaccine failures in these older age groups would lead to accumulation of susceptibles who cause epidemics in the future. Multiple dose measles vaccination strategies could reduce occurrence of these susceptibles thus averting the occurrence of epidemics and maintaining low measles transmission.

A two-pronged strategy was used in the provision of multiple doses of measles vaccine. The first variant of this strategy was that of a rapid and comprehensive "clean up" vaccination campaign targeted at all children aged 12-119 months (regardless of disease history or vaccination status) to clear this population of all susceptibles. This campaign was carried out over a two week period in early 1990. In the second variant of the strategy children who had had vaccination at 9 months of age at the city's static health facilities were given another single dose (revaccination) at any point between ages of 12 and 23 months at the same facilities. This second strategy was implemented over the rest of the project period from immediately after the campaign.

In Gweru routine vaccinations are indicated on child health cards and data on vaccinations are compiled monthly. From 1990 revaccination were also indicated on child health cards and figures on revaccinations were also complied monthly. Vaccinations applied during mass campaign of 1990 were indicated on child health cards. Children that did not have child health cards had new ones issued to them on which the campaign vaccination was indicated. Records compiled after the campaign indicated the number of children vaccinated in age classes 12-23, 24-59 and 60-119 months.

Gweru has had an active measles surveillance system since 1967. Measles cases are identified on the basis of a standard clinical case definition that is available to staff at all healthcare facilities. There are personnel who are assigned to investigate occurrence of unreported infectious diseases (including measles cases) within communities (active case search). Measles surveillance/investigation forms which have been in use indicate age at infection, gender, presenting/clinical features of disease, need for hospitalization or lack of it, treatment regime, outcome of illness (alive or dead), and occurrence of any other cases in relation to the identified case (which would also be investigated). Indication of vaccination status of measles cases was added to the form in January 1980. When the multiple dose vaccination effort was commenced in 1990 a slot was added on the surveillance form to indicate whether a case had had revaccination either during the campaign of 1990 or routine revaccination that followed the campaign or none. Information from surveillance forms is compiled monthly.

Bulawayo city was selected to partner the city of Gweru as a "control" at the inception of the multiple dose measles vaccination project in Gweru in 1990 for several reasons. These included: (a) Up till 1990 the vaccination practices in Bulawayo were similar to those of Gweru. Bulawayo city, like Gweru, had maintained high measles vaccination coverage rates for the vaccine applied at nine months of age and it had the capacity to maintain these rates during the project period 1990-96, (b) Structures for measles disease surveillance and monitoring of measles vaccinations in Bulawayo are similar to those of Gweru, and (c) The age structure of the populations in Gweru and Bulawayo were similar and so where the living conditions of the two populations.

The following comparisons were carried out: (a) Vaccination coverage rates for vaccine applied at nine months of age in Gweru and Bulawayo in the periods 1983-89 and 1990-96.

(b) Incidence rates of measles in Gweru and Bulawayo in the periods 1998-89 and 1990-96. (c) Incidence rates of vaccinated cases (vaccine failures) among children aged 10-119 months in both Gweru and Bulawayo cities in the period 1993-96. (d) Incidence rates of measles in children aged 60-119 months in both Gweru and Bulawayo in 1993-96.

The following analyses were carried out: (a) The student t test was used to compare means of normally distributed data, (b) The Kruskal – Wallis test was used to compare medians of non-normally distributed data, (c) The linear trend was determined using chi-square test for linear trend, (d) 95% confidence intervals were computed in order to indicate changes in the incidence rates, and (e) The cut off point for statistical significance was 5%.

FINDINGS

In Bulawayo in 1983-89 vaccine coverage rates for the vaccine applied at nine months of age were 77.0-93.0% (mean = 85.7, SD = 5.9) while in Gweru in the same period coverage rates were 72.0-92.0% (mean = 84.6, SD = 7.7). These coverage rates were not significantly different ($p = 0.736$). In Bulawayo in1990-96 vaccine coverage rates for the vaccine applied at nine months of age were 86.0-90.0% (mean = 89.0, SD = 1.8) while in Gweru in the same period they were 87.0-92.0% (mean = 89.7, SD = 1.7). These coverage rates were not significantly different ($p = 0.464$).

In 1990-96 in Gweru coverage rates for the second dose of measles vaccine applied to children at 12-23 months were 81-87% (mean = 82.4, SD = 2.1). In the mass vaccination campaign of 1990 in Gweru children aged 12-23, 24-59 and 60-119 months had vaccine coverage rates of 83.0%, 87% and 89% respectively.

In Bulawayo in 1983-89 measles incidence rates were 41.0-820.0/100 000 population (median = 254.0, $Q_1 = 79.0$, $Q_3 = 450.0$) while those in Gweru in the same period were151.0-450.0/100 000 population (median = 261.0, $Q_1 = 156.0$, $Q_3 = 400.0$). The incidence rates in the two cities were not significantly different ($p = 0.898$). Incidence rates in both Bulawayo and Gweru in 1983-89 significantly declined (Bulawayo: X^2 for linear trend = 446.04, $p < 0.001$ and Gweru: X^2 for linear trend = 88.83, $p < 0.001$) as shown in Figure 1. In 1990-96 measles incidence rates in Bulawayo were 19.0-313.0/100 000 population (median = 131.0, $Q_1 = 20.0$, $Q_3 = 193.0$) while those in Gweru were 9 to 29.0/100 000 population (median = 19.0, $Q_1 = 13.0$, $Q_3 = 22.0$). These incidence rates were significantly different ($p = 0.021$). Bulawayo city had measles epidemics in1992, 1993, 1994 and 1996 as shown in Figure 1.

The 121-2004 cases of measles (median = 1069.0, $Q_1 = 550.0$, $Q_3 = 1581.5$) aged 10-119 months reported in Bulawayo city in 1993-96 accounted for 98.6-99.9% (mean 99.1, SD 0.6) of all cases measles cases reported in that period. Of these cases some 58.0-64.0% (median = 58.5) had had vaccination against measles. In the same age group in the same period in Gweru 22-30 cases of measles (median = 25.5, $Q_1 = 23$, $Q_3 = 28.5$) were reported of whom 5-11cases (median 10.0) had had measles vaccination at 9 months of age. Incidence rates of vaccinated measles cases in the age group 10-119 months in

Bulawayo that relied solely on a vaccination programme that applied the vaccine at 9 months of age, Gweru may have avoided high occurrence of cases among older children aged >60 months on account of the vaccination campaign of 1990 which covered these children who were either revaccinated if they had had vaccination in infancy or received vaccination for the first time if they had not had vaccination before.

Although vaccination coverage rates for the vaccine applied at nine months of age were as high in Gweru as in Bulawayo in 1990-96, thus minimizing occurrence of unvaccinated cases in both cities in this period, the mass vaccination campaign of 1990 gave Gweru an opportunity to reach many susceptibles in the various age groups that were included in the campaign. This could partially explain the low measles transmission that occurred in Gweru and not in Bulawayo where a similar campaign was not carried out.

In conclusion, in 1983-89 in both Gweru and Bulawayo, at high vaccination coverage rates of single dose measles vaccine applied at nine months of age, measles transmission declined. Bulawayo, despite maintenance of high coverage rates of vaccine applied at nine months of age in 1990-96, had accumulation of vaccine failures in children aged 10-119 months and susceptibles (both vaccine failures and unvaccinated children) among older children aged 60 months and over that gave rise to epidemics after a period of declining and low transmission. In Gweru in 1990-96 application of multiple dose measles vaccination regime led to low level of measles transmission (compared to Bulawayo) by minimizing vaccine failures and cases among older children aged 60 months and over.

ACKNOWLEDGMENTS

This chapter is a revised version of an original paper published in the European Journal of Preventive Medicine (Marufu T, Siziya S, Tinago W. Comparison of Impact of Single Dose and Multiple Dose Measles Vaccination Strategies on Measles Transmission Patterns. Eur J Prev Med 2015;3:80-4) and the authors have obtained the permission from European Journal of Preventive Medicine to use this material.

REFERENCES

[1] Marufu T, Siziya S. Impact of multiple dose measles vaccination on measles transmission patterns in Gweru, Zimbabwe. J Trop Pediatr 2001; 47:335-8.

[2] Expanded Programme on Immunization. Measles control in the 1990s: Plan for action for global measles control. Geneva: WHO/EPI/GEN/92.3, 1992.

[3] Global Programme for Vaccines and Immunization. Immunization policy. Expanded programme on immunization. Geneva: WHO/EPI/GEN/95.3, 1995.

[4] Kambarami RA, Nathoo KJ, Nkrumah FK, Pirie GJ. Measles epidemic in Harare, Zimbabwe, despite high measles immunization coverage rates. Bull World Health Organ 1991; 69:213-9.

[5] Chen RT, Weierbach R, Bisoffi Z, Cutts F, Rhodes P, Ramaroson S, et al. A "post honeymoon period' measles outbreak in Muyinga sector, Burundi. Int J Epidemiol 1994; 23:185-93.

[6] Cutts F. Expanded programme on immunization. Measles control in the 1990s: Principles for next decade. Geneva: WHO/EPI/GEN/90.2, 1990.

[7] Coetzee N, Hussey GD, Visser G, Barron P, Keen A. The 1992 measles epidemic in Cape Town: A changing epidemiological pattern. S African Med J 1994; 84:145-9.

[8] Marufu T, Siziya S, Manyame B, Xaba E, Silape Z, Zimbizi P, et al. Questioning the level of efficacy of the measles vaccine that is in use in Zimbabwe. Cent Afr J Med 1995; 41:241-5.

[9] Expanded Programme on Immunization. Global measles strategy picks up pace. EPI Newsletter 1994; 16:3.

[10] Marufu T, Siziya S, Tshimanga S, Murugasampillay S, Mason E. Comparison of protection afforded by single measles vaccination and late revaccination schedules. E Afr Med J 1997; 74:777-9.

[11] Rosenthal SR, Clemens CJ. Two-dose measles vaccination schedules. Bull World Health Organ 1993; 71:421-8.

[12] Global Programme for Vaccines. Measles control in the 1990s: Final draft report for of GPV/CVI informal consultation on strategies to accelerate global measles control. Washington DC: EPI/WHO, 1994.

[13] Najwa A Khuri-Bulos. Measles in Jordan: a prototype of problems with measles in developing countries. Pediatr Infect Dis J 1997; 14:22-6.

SECTION THREE: COMPLICATED MEASLES AND MORTALITY

In: Measles
Editors: T. Marufu, S. Siziya et al.

ISBN: 978-1-63485-559-4

Chapter 9

FACTORS ASSOCIATED WITH SECULAR TRENDS IN MORTALITY ATTRIBUTED TO MEASLES

Tawanda Marufu[1,*], MB ChB, MSc,
Seter Siziya[2], BA (Ed), MSc, PhD
and Kaka Mudambo[3], MPH, PhD

[1]Liverpool JMU Centre for Public Health, Castle House, North Street, Liverpool, UK
[2]Department of Community Medicine, University of Zambia, Lusaka, Zambia and
[3]Department of Physiology, University of Zimbabwe, Harare, Zimbabwe

In this chapter we report on a retrospective study conducted in Gweru, Zimbabwe, that investigated the trend and its associated factors in measles mortality between 1967 and 1989. Measles and malnutrition surveillance data were analysed in SPSS version 8.0 using the Forward Stepwise Linear Regression method. Measles case fatality rates ranged from zero to 48.2% (median = 4.2, Q_1= 1.2, Q_3 =12.9) and they significantly linearly declined (slope = -1.686; 95% CI [-2.327, -1.044]; R^2 =59%). Rates of mortality among complicated measles cases (slope = 0.239, 95% CI [0.133, 0.345]) and rates of mortality from malnutrition among under-fives (slope= 0.065, 95% CI [0.031, 0.099]) independently

* Corresponding author: Tawanda Marufu, University of Zimbabwe College of Health Sciences, Box A 178, Avondale, Harare, Zimbabwe. E-mail: marufut@yahoo.com.

predicted (R^2=87%) measles case fatality rates. It was concluded that decline in rates of mortality among complicated measles cases, probably due to good management of such cases, and decline in rates of malnutrition among children aged <5 years may have contributed to the decline in measles case fatality rates.

INTRODUCTION

Recent studies have attributed major declines in measles mortality in Africa to supplementary measles immunization activities (SIAs) that were applied in1996 and after (1, 2). In the city of Gweru in Zimbabwe (population: 141,260, census of 2002) measles surveillance data seemed to indicate that mortality attributed to measles had consistently declined since the late 1960s, a decline that predates the supplementary immunization activities of the mid 1990s. We were curious to verify the decline in measles mortality in Gweru and, if the decline had occurred at all, to attempt to explain reasons for this occurrence. A retrospective study was carried out in Gweru to quantify changes in measles mortality in the period 1967-1989 and to explore factors associated with these changes. This paper reports on this study

OUR STUDY

Measles disease surveillance data for the period 1967-89 were analysed. Trends in measles case fatality rates were quantified. Association between measles case fatality rates and factors such as measles vaccination coverage rates, measles incidence rates, rates of complications among cases, nutritional status of children aged <5 years, etc. were explored.

Measles cases were identified through a surveillance system that recorded cases and deaths that were reported from the city's health centres and those reported from the community. Complicated measles cases were managed at the city's single infectious disease hospital. Data on measles cases and deaths were entered on line lists that indicated date of identification of a case, age at infection, gender, vaccination status, presenting features, whether admitted into hospital or not, treatment and outcome of illness (alive or dead). In Gweru, measles vaccinations have been applied to children at 9 months of age at static health facilities since 1971and records of vaccinations have been available since then.

The study used nutritional mortality data among under fives as a proxy for nutritional status of this age group. In Gweru, records on mortality attributed to nutritional deficiencies in children aged <5 years have been available since 1960. This data indicate date of death, age at death, gender and type of nutritional deficiency responsible for death.

Measles surveillance data and data on nutritional mortality in children aged <5 years were reviewed. The following were determined for each year: Measles case fatality rates, measles vaccination coverage rates, Measles incidence rates in the general population, measles incidence rates in children aged <23 months and incidence rates in children aged 60-119 months, rates of complications among cases, rates of respiratory complications among cases, rates of diarrhoeal complications among cases, rates of mortality among complicated cases, and nutritional mortality rates among children aged under five years. The data was entered into and analysed in SPSS version 8.0 for windows. The forward stepwise multiple linear regression analysis was used to determine independent predictors of measles case fatality rates. The probability of the F test for the variable to enter the model was set at 5% and to remove was 6%.

The following were limitations for the study: (a) Measles deaths cited in this study relate to immediate deaths attributed to acute disease and not post-measles deaths (3) that have been known to occur after the acute phase and are usually not recognized as measles deaths. This could have underestimated measles deaths that occurred in Gweru in the period under review, and (b) Phenomena such as over-crowding and intensive exposure that are said to affect severity of measles cases (2) were not examined in this study because the study relied on measles surveillance data where that information was not available.

FINDINGS

Variables that were examined in this study are indicated in table 1. In 1967-89 case fatality rates ranged from zero to 48.2% (median = 4.2, Q_1 = 1.2, Q_3 = 12.9) (see Table 1 and Figure 1). In this period case fatality rates significantly linearly declined (slope = -1.686, 95% CI [-2.327, -1.044]; R^2 = 59%). Major decline in case fatality rates occurred in 1967-79 after which low rates were recorded.

Table 1. Variables examined in the study

Year	Case fatality rates %	Vaccine coverage rates at 9 months of age (%)	Measles incidence rates in general population /100 000 population	Measles incidence rates in children aged <23 months /100 000 population	Measles Incidence rates in children aged 60-119 months /100 000 population	Rates of compli-cations among cases (%)	Rates of respiratory compli-cations (%)	Rates of diarrhea among cases (%)	Rates of mortality among complicated cases (%)	Nutritional mortality rates in under-fives /100 000 population
67	47.6	0	410	2609	235	27.2	17.4	4.9	96.3	216.1
68	37.7	0	260	2599	153	20.3	12.4	5.3	87.9	288.4
69	48.2	0	230	2135	168	40.8	32.6	0	98.2	446.4
70	25.2	0	121	2586	284	30.1	21.7	2.1	83.5	59.9
71	14.9	2	70	1482	337	26.3	21	1.8	72.9	18.5
72	5.2	16	110	2534	161	30.2	14.8	9.7	69.6	94.5
73	12.9	27	148	1810	154	30.7	12.3	16.9	27.8	40.2
74	6.3	29	220	2491	501	5.4	3.9	0.5	29.2	105.7
75	5.8	34	87	799	71	9.6	3.8	3.8	28.8	56.9
76	1.7	39	110	901	41	24.1	19	5.1	23.3	13.43
77	1.9	47	230	2342	510	25.5	18.6	6.1	10.7	32.2
78	42	56	148	689	114	22.5	19.7	1.4	11.2	51.6
79	4.8	63	316	1916	523	61.9	10.9	49.5	8.9	46.2
80	3.2	65	120	1189	200	54.8	11.1	30.2	11.9	88.2
81	1.7	73	80	1364	228	69.5	26.1	43.4	7.8	30.1

Year	Case fatality rates %	Vaccine coverage rates at 9 months of age (%)	Measles incidence rates in general population /100 000 population	Measles incidence rates in children aged <23 months /100 000 population	Measles Incidence rates in children aged 60-119 months /100 000 population	Rates of compli-cations among cases (%)	Rates of respiratory compli-cations (%)	Rates of diarrhea among cases (%)	Rates of mortality among complicated cases (%)	Nutritional mortality rates in under-fives /100 000 population
82	1.2	77	317	2393	353	8.2	3.3	3.3	15.3	25.3
83	2.6	72	400	3759	551	6.7	1.7	4.4	29.2	52.6
84	6.1	82	56	326	49	26.5	4.1	18.3	5.3	4.5
85	0.57	90	450	2464	1123	14.2	5.9	7.6	6.8	21.8
86	0	88	359	1549	926	12.6	2.5	7.8	0	29.8
87	0	92	261	1027	909	29.6	9.7	16.5	0	4
88	0.34	91	205	781	807	21.8	5.9	14.4	1.7	11.6
89	0	91	151	421	678	24.4	7.3	14	0	18.6
***Ran**										
*Min.	0	0	56.0	326	41	5.4	1.7	0	0	4
*Max.	48.2	92	4500	3759	1132	69.5	32.6	49.5	98.2	446.4
***Per c**										
Q_1	1.2	16	110	901	154	14.2	4.1	3.3	6.8	18.6
*Med	4.2	56	205	1810	284	25.5	11.1	6.1	15.3	40.2
Q_3	12.9	82	316	2491	551	30.2	19.0	16.5	69.6	88.2

* Ran= range, *Min = minimum, * Max = Maximum, *Perc = percentiles, *Med= median

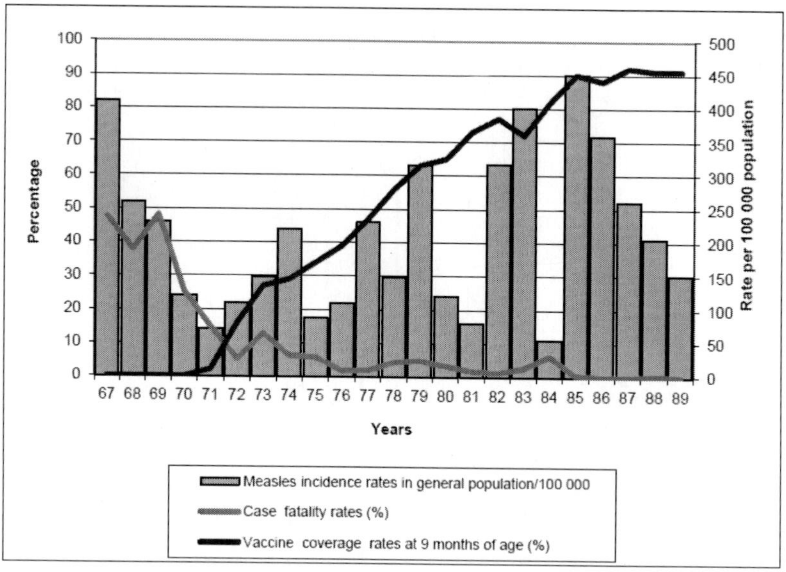

Figure 1. Measles case fatality rates, measles vaccine coverage rates and measles incidence rates in the general population in Gweru in 1967-1989.

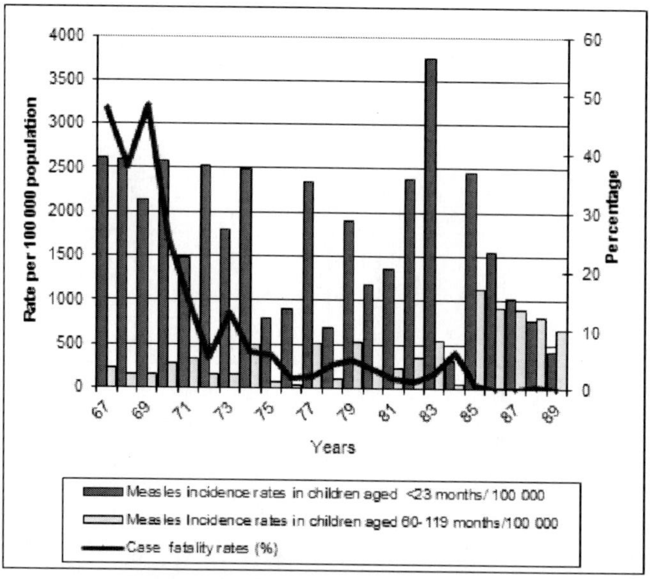

Figure 2. Measles case fatality rates, measles incidence rates in children aged <23 months and measles incidence rates in children aged 60-119 months in Gweru in 1967-1989.

Measles vaccination was commenced in 1971. In 1971-89 vaccine coverage rates were 0-92% (median=56, Q_1= 16, Q_3 = 82) (see Table 1 and Figure 1). In 1971-79 measles vaccine coverage rates were below 65%. Coverage rates of >80% were recorded in 1984-89. In 1967-89 measles incidence rates in the general population were 56-450/100 000 population (median=205, Q_1= 110, Q_3 = 316) (see Table 1 and Figure 1).

Incidence rates in children aged <23 months were, in 1967-89, 326-3759/100 000 population (median = 1810, Q_1 = 901, Q_3 = 2491) while those in children aged 60-119 months were 41-113/100 000 population (median=284, Q_1 = 110, Q_3 = 551) (see Table 1, Figure 2). Over most of the period under review incidence rates in children aged <23 months were higher than those of children aged 60-119 months up till 1988.

In 1967-89 rates of complications among measles cases were 5.4-69.5% (median = 25.5, Q_1=14.2, Q_3 = 30.2) as shown in Table 1 and Figure 3. Highest rates of complication of 61.9-69.5% were recorded in 1979-81. Among measles cases respiratory complications and diarrhoea accounted for 75.4-100% of all reported complications in the period under review (median = 87.3, Q_1 = 81.5, Q_3 = 95.1). In 1967-79 rates of respiratory complications and diarrhoea among measles cases were 3.8-32% (median =17.4, Q_1 =12.3, Q_3 = 19.7) and 0-49.5% (median = 4.9, Q_1 = 1.8, Q_3 = 6.1) respectively while in 1980-89 these were 1.7-26.1% (median = 5.9, Q_1 = 3.3, Q_3 = 9.7) and 3.3-43.4% (median =14.2, Q_1 = 7.6, Q_3 = 18.3) respectively.

In 1967-89 rates of mortality among complicated cases were 0-98.2% (median: 15.3, Q_1 = 15.3, Q_3 = 69.6) while rates of mortality from malnutrition in children aged <5 years were 4-446/100 000 population (median: 40.2, Q_1 =18.6, Q_3 = 88.2) (see Table 1, Figure 4). In the period under review rates of mortality among complicated cases significantly linearly declined (slope = -4.405; 95% CI [-5.499, -3.310]; R^2 = 77%) while mortality from malnutrition in children aged <5 years also significantly linearly declined (slope = -9.739; 95%CI [-15.225, -4.253]; R^2 = 39%) in the same period.

The constant term was not significant and was, therefore, excluded from further analysis. Results indicated that rates of mortality among complicated measles cases (slope = 0.239, 95% CI [0.133, 0.345]) and rates of mortality from malnutrition in underfives (slope = 0.065, 95% CI [0.031, 0.099]) were independent predictors of measles case fatality rates with an adjusted coefficient of determination of 86.7%. Variables that included rates of complications among cases, rates of respiratory complications among cases, rates of diarrhoeal complications among cases, measles incidence rates in the population, measles incidence rates in children aged <23 months, measles incidence rates in children aged 60-119 months, and measles vaccine coverage rates were not independent predictors of measles case fatality rates.

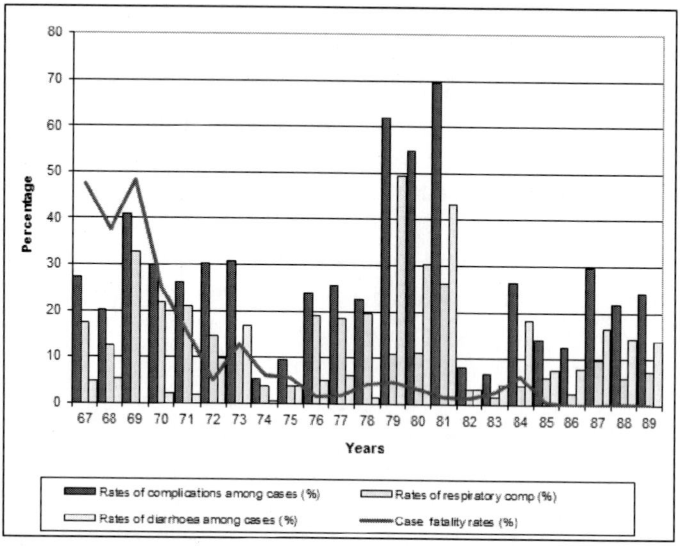

Figure 3. Measles case fatality rates, rates of complications among measles cases, rates of respiratory complications among measles cases and rates of diarrhoea among measles cases.

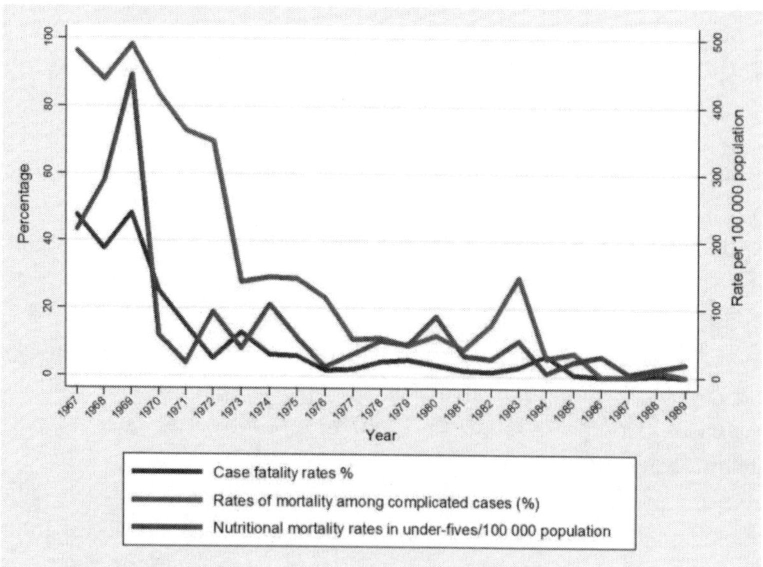

Figure 4. Measles case fatality rates, rates of mortality among complicated measles cases and nutritional mortality rates among children aged <5 yearsDiscussion

This study found that decline in rates of mortality among complicated measles cases and malnutrition mortality among children aged <5 years were both associated with the decline in measles case fatality rates. No significant associations were observed between measles vaccine coverage rates, measles incidence rates and rates of complications among cases on one hand and decline in measles case fatality rates on the other.

The current study found a significant association between rates of mortality among complicated cases (which declined over most of the period under review) and decline in measles case fatality rates. It is likely that improvements in management of measles cases may have reduced the rates of mortality among complicated cases. This observation is supported by the fact that: (a) Among measles cases, respiratory complications and diarrhoea are attended with higher case fatality rates than other complications and this is more so for respiratory complications than diarrhoea (4). This study found that respiratory complications and diarrhoea were predominant complications reported in the period under review. It was also found that higher rates of respiratory complications were recorded in 1967-79 than in 1980-89. However, despite the higher rates of respiratory complications in 1967-79, a major decline in measles case fatality rates occurred in the same period, and (b) Measles case fatality rates are highest in children aged <23 months (5). The current study found that measles incidence rates in that age group remained high up till 1987 and were higher than those of age group 60-119 months over most of the period under review. Despite this high occurrence of measles in children aged <23 months measles case fatality rates declined in 1967-89.

Although no direct measurement of quality of care of measles cases was carried out in this study, there have been long standing policies relating to management of measles cases in Gweru that indicate that adequate attention was given to care of complicated cases. Records show that all complicated cases were admitted into the infectious disease hospital. Since the mid to late 1960s as a matter of policy, over and above all therapies applied to complicated cases, vitamin A supplements were provided. Vitamin A is known to have an effect on survival of measles cases (4, 6). The importance of care of complicated cases is underlined by the observation that in most developing countries if measles deaths are to be reduced it would not be enough to rely on measles immunization alone. The majority of children infected with measles can be saved from death by improvements in case management and treatment of complications (5, 6). Findings of the current study seem to confirm this observation.

The current study found a significant association between rates of mortality from malnutrition in children aged <5 years (which declined in the period under review) and the decline in measles case fatality rates. Studies have found that communities with high rates of malnutrition have high measles case fatality rates (7, 8). It has, however, also been observed that despite this occurrence individual nutritional status is not a reliable predictor of mortality (9, 10). Thus the extent to which malnutrition contributes to incidence of infection and severity of infection is not clear or probably nonspecific (7). A large clinical controlled trial on effects of nutrition and medical care on morbidity and mortality from infectious diseases in children aged zero to three years was carried out in the Punjab, India. Analyses of growth rates, morbidity and mortality rates at different ages from this study showed benefits derived from both nutritional and medical care but did not show clearly which was greater (11). Despite the nonspecific nature of the relationship between malnutrition and infection, findings of the current study seem to suggest that it would be futile to have a programme solely directed at controlling measles without taking into account the nutritional status of children since level of nutrition would have a bearing on the survival of measles cases.

In conclusion, decline in mortality among complicated measles cases was probably due to good management of such cases, and decline in malnutrition among children aged <5 years may have led to a decline in measles case fatality rates in Gweru in the period 1967-1989. We would recommend that future studies explore and determine the quantity and quality of care required to reduce measles case fatality rates and how this same effort enmeshes with factors such as nutritional status of children.

ACKNOWLEDGMENTS

This chapter is a revised version of an original paper published in the Journal of Tropical Pediatrics (Marufu T, Siziya S, Mudambo K. Factors associated with secular trends in mortality attributed to measles in Gweru, Zimbabwe, in 1967-1989. J Trop Ped 2007; 54: 114-9) and the authors have obtained the permission from Journal of Tropical Pediatrics to use this material.

REFERENCES

[1] Biellik R, Madema S, Taole A, Kutsulukuta A, Allies E, Eggers R, et al. First 5 years of measles elimination in southern Africa: 1996-2000.Lancet 2002; 359: 1564-8.

[2] Otten M, Kezaala R, Fall A, Masresha B, Martin R, Cairns L, et al. Public health impact of accelerated measles control in the WHO African Region 2000-03. Lancet 2005; 366: 832-9.

[3] Markowitz LE, Orenstein WA.Measles vaccines. Pediatr Clin North Am 1990; 37: 603-25.

[4] Division of Diarrhoeal and Acute Respiratory Diseases Control, Global programme for Vaccines and Immunization and Expanded Programme on Immunization. Clinical research on treatment of measles: report of a meeting. Banjul, Gambia. 3-5 November 1993.

[5] Foster SO, McFarland DA, John AM. Measles. In: Jamison DT, Mosley WH, Measham AR, Bobadilla JL, eds. Disease control priorities in developing countries. New York: Oxford University Press, 1993: 161–87.

[6] Expanded programme on Immunization. Measles control – a global battle in progress, recommendations for the remainder of the decade. Geneva: World Health Organization, Update, 1993.

[7] Rodrigues LC. EPI target diseases: measles, tetanus, polio, tuberculosis, pertussis, and diphtheria. In: Feachem RG, Jamison DT, eds. Disease and mortality in sub-Saharan Africa. Oxford: Oxford University Press, 1991: 173-89.

[8] Singh J1, Sharma RS, Verghese T. Measles mortality in India: a review of community based studies. J Commun Dis 1994; 26(4): 203-14.

[9] Aaby P, Coovadia H. Severe measles: a reappraisal of the role of nutrition, overcrowding and virus dose. Med Hypotheses 1985; 18: 93-112.

[10] Koster FT, Curlin GC, Aziz KM, Haque A. Synergistic impact of measles and diarrhoea on nutrition and mortality in Bangladesh. Bull World Health Organ 1981; 59: 901-8.

[11] Kielmann AA, Taylor CE, Parker RL. The Narangwal Nutrition Study: a summary review. Am J Clin Nutr 1978; 31: 2040-57.

In: Measles
Editors: T. Marufu, S. Siziya et al.

ISBN: 978-1-63485-559-4

Chapter 10

FACTORS ASSOCIATED WITH MEASLES COMPLICATIONS

Tawanda Marufu[1,*], MB ChB, MSc, Seter Siziya[1], BA (Ed), MSc, PhD, Mufuta Tshimanga[1], MD, MPH, Shiva Murugasampillay[2], MBBS, MSc, Elizabeth Mason[2], MBChB, MSc and Boniface Manyame[3], MB ChB, MPH

[1]University of Zimbabwe Medical School, Harare, Zimbabwe,
[2]WHO Country Office, Harare, Zimbabwe and
[3]UNICEF Country Office, Harare, Zimbabwe

A cross sectional study was conducted to investigate factors associated with complications or death among measles cases. The study that was conducted in health facilities in the city of Gweru, Zimbabwe, had a total of 637 measles cases randomly selected from measles surveillance data. Main outcome measures of the study were:(a) Associations of respiratory complications and diarrhoea with death among complicated cases; (b) associations of age at infection, gender of cases and vaccination status of cases with occurrence of either respiratory complications or diarrhoea or death among measles cases. Among cases with respiratory complications, 22 (29%) had died, while 5 (5%) had died

* Corresponding author: Tawanda Marufu, University of Zimbabwe College of Health Sciences, Box A 178, Avondale, Harare, Zimbabwe. E-mail: marufut@yahoo.com.

among those with diarrhoea (OR = 7, 95% CI [3, 22], $p < 0.001$). On rates of respiratory complications among cases, age groups 24-59 and 60+ months were protective by 57% (95% CI [11, 79%]) and 76% (95% CI [52, 88%]) respectively compared to the age group <24 months, and vaccination was protective by 42% (95% CI [2, 65%]) compared to those unvaccinated. Concerning rates of diarrhoea among cases, the age group 60+ months was protective by 80% (95% CI [62, 89%]) compared to age group <60 months, while vaccination was protective by 64% (95% CI [42, 77%]) compared to those unvaccinated. With respect to rates of mortality among cases, age was protective by 6% (95% CI [3, 9%]) for every year older. It was concluded that: (a) the risk of death was higher in cases with respiratory complications than diarrhoea; (b) the risk of complications and death was inversely related to age at infection and older age groups were protective against occurrence of complications or death; (c) the risk of complications was higher in unvaccinated cases and vaccination was protective against occurrence of complications.

INTRODUCTION

The city of Gweru in Zimbabwe has a population of 124,735 (1992 Census). In this city an investigation was carried out to identify factors associated with measles complications or death in order to workout modalities for reducing their occurrence. This paper presents the findings of that investigation.

OUR STUDY

A cross-sectional study that used surveillance data for the period 1980-89 compared measles cases with complications or had died with those without complications or had not died. In Gweru, measles cases and deaths were identified through a surveillance system which recorded cases and deaths that were reported from the city's health centres and those reported through active case searches in the community. Data on the measles cases and deaths were entered on line lists which indicated date of identification of a case, age at infection, gender, vaccination status, presenting features, whether admitted into hospital or not and outcome of illness (alive or dead).

Measles surveillance data for the period January 1980 through December 1989 were reviewed. It was decided that all deaths that had occurred in that period be included in the study. Measles cases that had had complications in that period were estimated at about thirty per cent. Based on this estimate on the occurrence of complications among measles cases, the optimal sample size (at 95% confidence level) was 620 using Stat-Calc of EPI-info version 5. A one in four systematic sampling procedure was used to select participants into the study from the surveillance line lists.

Data analysis was conducted as follows: (a) Respiratory complications and diarrhoea were correlated with rates of deaths among complicated cases and; (b) age at infection, gender and vaccination status of cases were correlated with rates of occurrence of respiratory complications, diarrhoea and deaths among cases. Initial analysis entailed bivariate analysis of age, gender and vaccination status and either rates of respiratory complications or diarrhoea or deaths. Further analysis to adjust for possible confounding variables entailed logistic regression analysis of age, gender and vaccination status on rates of either respiratory complications or diarrhoea or deaths among cases.

Limitations of the study included: complications and deaths cited in this study are immediate complications and deaths attributed to acute measles and not delayed complications (1) or post-measles deaths (2, 3) which may not have been recognized as measles complications or deaths after the acute measles episode. Phenomena such as overcrowding and intensive exposure that are said to affect severity of measles cases (4, 5) were not examined in this study because the study relied on measles surveillance data where that information was not available. Malnutrition is said to be associated with the occurrence of complications among measles cases (1). This association was not examined in this study.

FINDINGS

Six hundred and thirty seven (637) cases of measles were enrolled into the study. One hundred and three cases (6.2%), 93 (14.6%), 15.4 (24.2%) and 287 (45.1%) were aged 0-11, 12-23, 24-59 and 60+ months respectively. There were 352 (55.3%) males and 285 females. Three hundred and thirty five (52.6%) cases had been vaccinated against measles while 302 (47.4%) had not had vaccination. Twenty eight (4.4%) of the cases in the sample had died.

Two hundred and nine cases in the sample had complications. Among the complicated cases, 76 (36.4%) had had respiratory complications while 10 (52.6%) had had diarrhoea. Another 23(11.0%) cases had other complications which included malnutrition, stomatitis, encephalitis, and otitis media. Among the 76 cases with respiratory complications, 22 (28.9%) had died while six (5.5%) had also died among the 10 cases with diarrhoea. The difference between occurrence of deaths among cases with respiratory complications and diarrhoea was significant (OR =7 (95% CI [3, 22], $p < 0.001$). No deaths occurred among cases with other complications.

In the age groups 0-11, I 2-23, 24-59 and 60+ months, rates of respiratory complications declined from the order of 23.3% to 5.9% as shown in Table 1. The declining trend in age-specific rates of respiratory complications was statistically significant (χ^2 for trend = 31.35, df = 3, $p < 0.001$). Among the 76 cases with respiratory complications, 44 (57.9%) were males while 32 were females. There was no significant association between gender and rates of respiratory complications among cases (χ^2 Yates corrected = 0.73, df = 1, p = 0.391). Among the 335 vaccinated cases in the sample 28 (8.4%) had respiratory complications while 48 (15.9%) of the 302 unvaccinated cases also had respiratory complications. There was a significant association between vaccination status and rates of respiratory complications among cases (χ^2 Yates corrected = 7.88, df = 1, p = 0.005).

Table 1. Age-specific rates of respiratory complications among measles cases

Age in months	With respiratory complications n (%)	No respiratory complications n (%)	Total
0-11	24 (23.3)	79 (76.6)	103
12-23	20 (21.5)	73 (78.5)	93
24-59	15 (9.7)	139 (90.3)	154
60+	17 (5.9)	270 (94.1)	287

Table 2. Age-Specific rates of diarrhoea among measles cases

Age in months	With diarrhoea n (%)	No diarrhoea n (%)	Total
0-11	33 (32.0)	70(68.0)	103
12-23	25 (26.9)	68 (73.1)	93
24-59	32 (20.8)	122 (79.2)	154
60+	20 (7.0)	267 (93.0)	287

A logistic regression analysis of age, gender and vaccination status on rates of respiratory complications showed that age groups 24-59 and 60+ months were protective by 57% (95% CI [11, 79%]) and 76% (95% CI [52, 88%]) respectively compared to the age group <24 months, and vaccination was protective by 42% (95% CI [2, 65%]) compared to the unvaccinated against occurrence of respiratory complications among cases.

In the age groups 0-11, 12-23, 24-59 and 60+ months, rates of diarrhoea declined from 32.0% to 7.0% as shown in Table 2. The declining trend in age-specific rates of diarrhoea was statistically significant (χ^2 for trend =44.38, df = 3, $p < 0.001$). Among 352 males in the sample, 57 (16.2%) had diarrhoea while among 285 females, 53 (18.6%) had had the same complication. There was no association between gender and rates of diarrhoea among cases (χ^2 Yates corrected=0.48, df = 1, p = 0.489). Among the 335 vaccinated cases in the sample, 34 (10.1%) had diarrhoea while among the 302 unvaccinated cases 76 (25.2%) had the same complication. Association between vaccination status and rates of diarrhoea was significant (χ^2 Yates corrected = 24.03, df= 1, $p < 0.001$).

A logistic analysis of age, gender and vaccination status diarrhoea among cases showed that age group 60+ months was protective by 80% (95% CI [62, 89%]) compared to <60 months age group while vaccination was protective by 64% (95% CI [42, 77%]) compared to non-vaccination.

In the age groups 0-11, 12-23, 24-59 and 60+ months deaths had occurred in the order of 13(12.6%), 13(14.0%), one (0.6%) and one (0.3%) respectively. The declining trend in age-specific mortality rates was significant (χ^2 for trend = 42. 73, df = 3, $p < 0.001$). Of the 28 measles deaths in the sample 16 were males while 12 were females. Among the 352 males enrolled into the survey, sixteen deaths represented 4.5% of this gender while twelve deaths among 285 females represented 4.2% of that gender. The gender-specific mortality rates were not significant (χ^2 =0.01, df = 1, p = 0.991). Among the 28 measles deaths, eight had been vaccinated against measles while 20 had not. Among the 335 vaccinated cases eight (2.3%) died while 20 (6.6%) of the 302 unvaccinated cases had also died (χ^2 Yates corrected = 5.16, df = 1, p = 0.016). Logistic regression analysis of age, gender and vaccination status on rates of deaths among cases showed that only age was protective by 6% (95% CI [3, 9%]) for every year older.

DISCUSSION

The spectrum of complications found in the current study confirms findings of studies from other developing countries. In these countries the major complications were pneumonia, croup and diarrhoea. Other complications included malnutrition, otitis media, severe stomatitis and neurological problems (1, 6, 7).

Studies carried out elsewhere found that respiratory complications and diarrhoea were attended with higher mortality than other complications among cases and also that cases with respiratory complications had a higher mortality than those with diarrhea (l, 7). In a measles epidemic in Harare, Zimbabwe, in which 20 cases died, pneumonia was the most frequent complication associated with death (11 cases) followed by diarrhoea with dehydration (6 cases) (7). A study in Afghanistan which looked at 784 measles cases admitted in a Kabul hospital found that respiratory complications including bronchopneumonia and croup were the commonest causes of death followed by encephalitis and gastroenteritis (8). Case fatality rates of 20-46%, 7-40% and 25% were reported among hospitalized measles cases with pneumonia, croup and diarrhoea respectively (1). Findings of the current study concur with those of previous studies where it was found that respiratory complications and diarrhoea were associated with deaths among cases and that this was more so for cases with respiratory complications than diarrhoea.

Studies have shown that the risk of serious measles complications is higher in young children and adults (3, 9). In a measles epidemic in Harare, Zimbabwe, it was found that among cases admitted into hospital, rates of all major complications (diarrhoea with dehydration, pneumonia, croup and convulsions) declined with age, with higher rates of complications among the young age groups of 23 months of age and under (7). In a measles outbreak in Rwanda reported age-specific case fatality rates decreased with age: 0-8 months, 3%; 9-23 months, 1.4%; 24-59 months, 1%; and 60 months and older, 0.5% (2). In Niakhar, Senegal, a major increase in measles vaccination which occurred between 1987 and 1990 saw the mean age at infection increase from four to seven years. The change in the age structure was said to have accounted for a 20% decline in measles case fatality rate (10). This change in age at infection has been observed in many countries with high vaccination coverage rates and the decline in measles mortality that has been observed in these countries has partially been attributed to this change in the age structure among measles cases (11). Findings of the current study confirm those of other studies where it was found that occurrence of respiratory complications, diarrhoea and deaths among cases declined with age and that increase in age at infection was protective against their occurrence.

In this study, it was found that the rate of complications among the vaccinated cases was significantly lower than among the unvaccinated. This contradicts the finding in a study in Harare, Zimbabwe, where the rate of complications was significantly higher among immunized cases than among those that were not (7). It would seem that this finding in Harare may have been influenced by factors such as a high prevalence of undernutrition among cases aged under fifteen years which is thought to have contributed to the severity of measles in that study (7). Studies that have been carried out in the general childhood population, not just among measles cases, have found measles vaccination protective against morbidity and mortality associated with pneumonia and diarrhoea. A case-control study to determine whether measles vaccination is associated with reduced mortality rate in rural Bangladeshi children (10-60 months of age) found that measles vaccine was associated with a 36% reduction in the overall rate of death and a 22% reduction in the rate of acute lower respiratory infection-related deaths (12, 13). In a study by Feachem and Koblinsky (14), it was estimated that measles immunization at the ages of 9-11 months, with coverage of 45-90% can avert 44-64% of measles cases, 0.6-3.8% of diarrhoea episodes, and 6-26% of diarrhoea deaths among children under five years of age. Although the current study did not look at the protection afforded the general childhood population against pneumonia and diarrhoea through vaccination, its findings seem to support those of other studies where it has been observed that vaccination is protective against these conditions.

Some studies found that vaccination was directly protective against occurrence of mortality among cases (3). A study from Zambia found that case fatality rates in vaccinated cases was 6.4% while that in unvaccinated cases was 17%. This same study observed that while measles vaccine cannot prevent infection it can reduce the severity of infection (15). A study in Senegal found that vaccinated children who contracted measles had significantly lower case fatality rate than unvaccinated children with measles and concluded that vaccination contributes to lower mortality indirectly through less severe infection for vaccinated cases (10). A study in Guinea-Bissau had similar findings and conclusions (16). In the current study, although in bivariate analysis it was found that vaccination was protective against occurrence of mortality, on logistic regression analysis of age, gender and vaccination status on rates of mortality among cases only age was protective. Vaccination status may, therefore, have been confounded by age or gender and thus may not have a direct influence on occurrence of mortality among cases. Findings of the current study therefore contradict findings of studies indicated above in that no relationship was found between vaccination status and occurrence of mortality among cases.

Review studies (10, 15, 16) have equated mild measles disease (reduced severity) with a lower case fatality rate which has been observed in vaccinated children. In these studies the role of complications in causing mortality is not explicit when it has been observed that most measles deaths are attributed to complications (12). Findings of the current study seem to suggest that vaccination makes measles disease mild directly through protection against occurrence of complications and indirectly through increasing age at infection (11) which was also found to be protective against occurrence of complications and deaths. However, the suggestion that vaccination could make the measles disease mild contradicts the observation that many cases of measles in persons with a history of vaccination are typical and severe, and occurrence of milder measles in previously vaccinated persons may represent one end of a spectrum of measles illness, independent of vaccination (3).

The current study found no association between gender and occurrence of respiratory complications, diarrhoea and deaths among measles cases. Studies in Bangladesh and India found excess measles mortality in females (17, 18). Studies in Africa have not shown these gender mortality differences. It has, thus, been suggested that the differences that have been observed could be due to gender-specific patterns of child care and response to illness rather than biological difference between sexes (2).

In conclusion, the current study found that: (a) the risk of death was higher in cases with respiratory complications than those with diarrhoea; (b) the risk of measles complications or death was inversely related to age at infection and older age groups were protective against occurrence of complications or death; (c) the risk of respiratory complications and diarrhoea was higher in unvaccinated cases, and vaccination was protective against the occurrence of these complications.

ACKNOWLEDGMENTS

This chapter is a revised version of an original paper published in the East African Medical Journal (Marufu T, Siziya S, Tshimanga M, Murugasampillay S, Mason E, Manyame B. Factors associated with measles complications in Gweru, Zimbabwe. East African Med J 2001; 78:135-8) and the authors have obtained the permission from East African Medical Journal to use this material.

REFERENCES

[1] Division of Diarrhoeal and Acute Respiratory Disease Control, Global programme for Vaccines and Immunization and Expanded Programme on Immunization. Clinical research on treatment of measles: Report of a meeting. Banjul, Gambia. 3-5 November, 1993. Geneva: WHO/CDR/95.15 and WHO/EPI/GEN/95.07, 1993.

[2] Foster SO, McFarland DA, John AM. Measles. In: Jamison DT, Mosley WH, Measham AR, Bobadilla JL, eds. Disease control priorities in developing countries. New York: Oxford University Press, 1993:161–87.

[3] Makowiwitz LE, Orenstein WA. Measles vaccines. Pediatr Clin North Am 1990; 37: 603-25.

[4] Aaby P. Malnutrition and overcrowding/intensive exposure in severe measles infection: review of community studies. Rev Infect Dis 1988; 10: 478-91.

[5] Aaby P, Bukh J, Lisse IM, da Silva MC. Further community studies on the role of overcrowding and intensive exposure on measles mortality. Rev Infect Dis 1988; 10: 474-7.

[6] Rodrigues LC. EPI target diseases: measles, tetanus, polio, tuberculosis, pertussis and diphtheria. In: Feachem RG, Jamison DT, eds. Disease and mortality in Sub-Saharan Africa. Oxford: Oxford University Press, 1991: 173-89.

[7] Kambarami RA, Nathoo KJ, Nkrumah FK, Pirie GJ. Measles epidemic in Harare, Zimbabwe, despite high measles immunization coverage rates. Bull World Health Organ 1991; 69: 213-9.

[8] Arya LS, Taana I, Tahiri C, Saidali A, Singh M. Spectrum of complications of measles in Afghanistan: a study of 784 cases. J Trop Med Hyg 1987; 90: 117-22.

[9] Cutts FT. The immunological basis for immunization No.7: Measles expanded programme on immunization. Geneva: WHO/ EPI/GEN/93.17, 1993.

[10] Samb B, Aaby P, Whittle H, Seek AM, Simondon F. Decline in measles case fatality ratio after the introduction of measles immunization in rural Senegal. Am J Epidemiol 1997; 145: 51-7.

[11] Global Programme for Vaccines and Immunization. Immunization policy. Expanded programme on immunization. Geneva: WHO/EPI/GEN/95.3, 1995.

[12] Markowitz LE, Nieburg P. The burden of acute respiratory infection due to measles in developing countries and the potential impact of measles vaccine. Rev Infect Dis 1991; 13(Suppl 6): S555-61.

[13] Clemens JD, Stanton BF, Chakraborty J, Chowdhury S, Rao MR, Ali M, Zimicki S, Wojtyniak B. Measles vaccination and childhood mortality in rural Bangladesh. Am J Epidemiol 1988; 128: 1330-9.

[14] Feachem RG, Koblinsky MA. Interventions for the control of diarrhoeal diseases among young children: measles immunization. Bull World Health Organ 1983; 61: 641-52.

[15] Oshitani H, Mpabalwani M, Kasolo F, Mizuta K, Luo NP, Bhat GJ, et al. Measles infection in hospitalized children in Lusaka, Zambia. Ann Trop Paediatr 1995; 15: 167-72.

[16] Aaby P, Bukh J, Leerhøy J, Lisse IM, Mordhorst CH, Pedersen IR. Vaccinated children get milder measles infection: A community study from Guinea-Bissau. J Infect Dis 1986; 154: 858-63.

[17] Bhuiya A, Wojtyniak B, D'Souza S, Nahar L, Shaikh K. Measles case fatality among the under-fives: a multivariate analysis of risk factors in a rural area of Bangladesh. Soc Sci Med 1987; 24: 439-43.

[18] Chand P, Rai RN, Chawla U, Tripathi KC, Datta KK. Epidemiology of measles--a thirteen years prospective study in a village. J Commun Dis 1989; 21: 190-9.

In: Measles
Editors: T. Marufu, S. Siziya et al.
ISBN: 978-1-63485-559-4

Chapter 11

SECULAR CHANGES IN RATES OF RESPIRATORY COMPLICATIONS AND DIARRHOEA AMONG MEASLES CASES

Tawanda Marufu**, MB ChB, MSc and
Seter Siziya, BA (Ed), MSc, PhD
Department of Community Medicine,
University of Zimbabwe Medical School, Harare, Zimbabwe

It has been observed that the occurrence of respiratory complications and diarrhoea among measles cases has changed over time but this change has not been quantified. A study was carried out in the city of Gweru, Zimbabwe, to quantify these changes. Rates of respiratory complications and diarrhoea among measles cases were determined in each year for the period 1968–89. It was found that mean rates of respiratory complications and diarrhoea during 1968–78 were 17.2% (95% CI [11.6, 22.8]) and 5.2% (95% CI [0, 11]) respectively while during 1979–89, mean rates of respiratory complications and diarrhoea were 6.5% (95% CI [1, 12.1]) and 16.4% (95% CI [10.1, 22.0]) respectively. Analysis of variance (ANOVA) to determine the main effects and the interaction showed that the main effects were not statistically significant ($F = 0.01$, $df_{1.2} = 1{,}40$, $p = 0.935$; and $F = 0.13$, $df_{1.2}=1{,}40$, $p=0.725$ respectively). Meanwhile the interaction term of complications and period was statistically significant ($F = 15.7$, $df._{1.2} =$

* Corresponding author: Tawanda Marufu, University of Zimbabwe College of Health Sciences, Box A 178, Avondale, Harare, Zimbabwe. E-mail: marufut@yahoo.com.

1,40, $p < 0.001$). It was concluded that a change in rates of respiratory complications and diarrhoea had occurred among measles cases. It is suggested that the increase in vaccination coverage in 1979–89 and the shift in age at infection to older age groups in the same period may have brought about this change through selective suppression of respiratory complications among measles cases.

INTRODUCTION

Measles complications, particularly pneumonia, croup, and diarrhoea, are associated with high case fatality rates (1, 2). In the City of Gweru, Zimbabwe, it had been observed that the occurrence of respiratory complications (pneumonia, croup, and tracheitis) and diarrhoea among measles cases had changed but this had not been quantified. A study was carried out in this city to quantify this change and to explain it.

OUR STUDY

Measles surveillance data for the period 1968-89 were analysed. These data were used in this study because they contain details on the occurrence of complications among measles cases. Measles surveillance data prior to 1968 do not have this information.

Gweru is the largest city in Zimbabwe, with a population of 124,735 (1992 census). Measles cases and deaths are identified through a surveillance system which records cases and deaths that are reported from the city's health centres and those reported through activity case searches in the community. Complicated cases are managed at the city's single infectious disease hospital. Data on measles cases and deaths are entered on line lists which indicate date of identification of a case, age at infection, gender, vaccination status, presenting features, whether admitted into hospital or not and outcome of illness (alive or dead).

Measles surveillance data (line list of cases) for the period 1968-1989 were reviewed. All cases of measles that had had complications were included in the study. Rates of occurrence of all complications, and those of diarrhoea and respiratory complications, were determined among cases. Analysis of variance (ANOVA) was used to determine the significance of the main effects and of the interaction term.

The study's limitation is that complications cited in the current study are immediate complications attributed to acute measles and not delayed complications (2, 3) which may not have been recognized as being measles-associated after the acute episode.

FINDINGS

In the period under review the spectrum of measles complications included pneumonia, diarrhoea, croup, tracheitis, malnutrition, otitis media, tonsillitis, stomatitis, and encephalitis. The rates of all complications among cases were in the range 5.4-69.5% (median = 25, $Q_1 = 14.5$, $Q_3 = 31.5$) in the period 1968-89. Other complications, excluding respiratory complications and diarrhoea, were in the range 0-14.6% (median = 2.0, $Q_1 = 1.6$, $Q_3 = 5.3$) among measles cases in the same period.

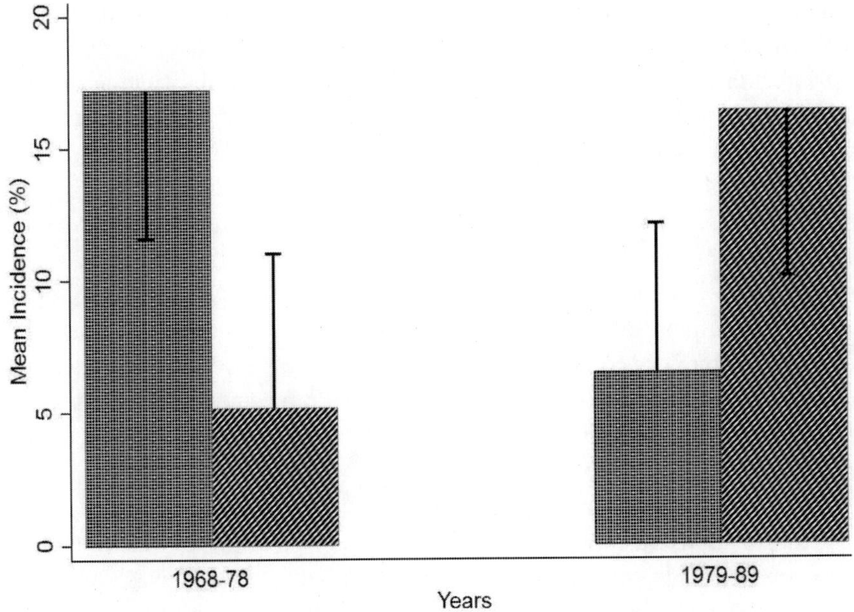

Figure 1. Mean rates of respiratory complications (filled squares) and diarrhea (hatched squares) among measles cases for the period 1968-78 and 1979-89.

In the period 1968-78 the mean rates of respiratory complications and diarrhoea among cases were 17.2% (95% CI [11.6-22.8%]) and 5.2% (95% CI [0, 11%]) respectively while in the period 1979-89 the mean rates of respiratory complications and diarrhoea were 6.5% (95% CI [1-12.1%]) and 16.4% (95% CI [10.1-22.0%]). Figure 1 shows the mean rates of respiratory complications and diarrhoea among cases in the two periods 1968-78 and 1979-89. The main effects of 'period' and 'complications' were not statistically significant ($F = 0.01$, $df_{1.2} = 1,40$, $p = 0.935$ and $F = 0.13$, $df_{1.2} = 1,40$, $p = 0.725$ respectively). However, the interaction between 'rates of complications' and 'period' was statistically significant ($F = 15.7$, $df_{1.2} = 1,40$, $p < 0.001$).

DISCUSSION

Measles complications seen in the present study are unlike those associated with measles infection in developed countries. In these countries the commonly cited complications are otitis media (7-9%) pneumonia (1-6%), post-infection encephalitis (1/1000-1/2000 cases) and sub-acute sclerosing pan-encephalitis (1/100 000 cases) (2, 4). The spectrum of complications seen in the current study confirm findings of studies from other developing countries. In these countries the major complications are pneumonia, croup, and diarrhoea. Other complications include malnutrition, otitis media, severe stomatitis, and neurological problems (3, 5, 6).

A study that looked at occurrence of severe measles (respiratory complications, diarrhoea, and deaths) among 637 cases in Gweru found that the risk of respiratory complications and diarrhoea was inversely related to age and that age groups 24-59 and 60+ months were protected against occurrence of respiratory complications by 57% and 76% respectively relative to age groups <23 months. Only the age group 60+ months was protected against occurrence of diarrhoea by 80% compared with age groups <59 months. Also, the risk of both respiratory complications and diarrhoea was higher in unvaccinated cases than in the vaccinated and vaccination was protective against the occurrence of respiratory complication and diarrhoea by 42% and 64% respectively compared to non-vaccination (7). From the findings of that study, it would seem that changes in age at infection and vaccination status of cases would also effect changes in rates of respiratory complications and diarrhoea among cases. Thus increase in vaccination coverage, which usually leads to an increase in the proportion of vaccinated measles cases and a shift in age at infection towards older age groups (8-10), would lead to a change in rates of either respiratory complications or diarrhoea among cases. To support this argument an attempt is made to explain the change in rates of respiratory complications and diarrhoea observed in the current study using findings of the study (7) cited above and other studies.

In the absence of vaccination or at low vaccination coverage, measles predominantly afflicts young age groups (3, 10). Under these conditions respiratory complications are the commonest among measles cases, presumably due to the fact that young children are prone to respiratory tract infections (which are inversely related to age) and that the measles virus (and superinfection that arises from its effects) affects predominantly the respiratory tree (3, 11, 12). In the current study this would have been the case in the period 1968-78 when rates of respiratoratory complications were higher than diarrhoea among cases. In Gweru in this period, vaccination coverage was low and measles occurred predominantly in children aged less than 23 months (13). Studies carried out in areas with either low vaccination rates or where measles predominantly afflicts the young have found that rates of respiratory complications are higher than those of diarrhoea among cases, as found in the current study in the period 1968-78. In a hospital study in Malaysia, where 85 percent of admitted cases were not immunized against measles (median age of cases was 12 months) the main complications were pneumonia (74.1%) and diarrhoea (38.1%) (14). A study in Afghanistan which looked at 784 cases of measles admitted into a Kabul hospital found that bronchopneumonia was the commonest complication (85%) followed by enteritis (30.2%) and croup (22%). In this study 73.6% of children (4 months-12 years) were below 3 years, with most cases in the 1-2 years age group (15).

In Gweru, a sharp increase in vaccination coverage which occurred after inception of the Expanded Programme on Immunization (EPI) after 1979 occasioned a shift of measles disease towards older age groups (24+ months) and an increase in the proportion of vaccinated cases (13, 16). This would have led to suppression of occurrence of respiratory complications, particularly from changes in age, which, as found in the study in Gweru (cited above), have been shown to have a bigger protective effect than vaccination (7). A study in Senegal found that respiratory complications were more common in secondary cases infected by an index case with respiratory complications than by an index case without respiratory complications, suggesting that severe cases give rise to further severe cases (17). It could be that in Gweru, as respiratory complications were suppressed through changes in age at infection and vaccination, their occurrence would have been further curtailed through generation of fewer secondary cases, as described in the study from Senegal. Suppression of respiratory complications would have left diarrhoea as the prominent complication. Further still, prominence of diarrhoea would have been strengthened by the fact that, although like respiratory complications diarrhoea could be suppressed by vaccination, it required a bigger shift in age at infection among cases for changes in age at infection to suppress its occurrence since (as shown in the study (7) in Gweru) only the age group 60+ months (and not the lower age groups) was protective against its occurrence. It would seem that increase in vaccination and the consequent change in age at infection which occurred after 1979 would have had a selective suppression of respiratory complications with the result that rates of diarrhoea among cases were higher than those of respiratory complications, as found in the current study. In an epidemic which occurred in 1988 in a community with vaccination coverage rates of 83% in Harare, Zimbabwe, where a shift of disease to older age groups was in progress, it was found that among the 1399 hospitalized cases, diarrhoea with dehydration accounted for 29% of cases, respiratory complications 26%, and convulsions 1%. Findings of this study seem to confirm those of the current study for the period 1979-89 in that rates of diarrhoea were greater than those of respiratory complications among measles cases.

Some studies have shown that overcrowding, intensity of exposure (18, 19) and malnutrition (3) are associated with occurrence of severe measles and thus could affect rates of complications among measles cases. In the absence of studies on these factors in Gweru, the extent to which such factors would have influenced changes in the rates of respiratory complications and diarrhoea among cases in the period under review is not clear.

In the city of Gweru mortality attributed to measles has been declining since 1967. In the period 1980-89 fewer deaths, compared to the earlier period, were reported (13). Respiratory complications, particularly pneumonia and croup, are associated with higher mortality rates among cases than diarrhea (2, 3). The current study has shown that in the period 1979 and after, the rates of respiratory complications among measles cases had declined. This would suggest that the decline in measles mortality rate after 1980 could partially be attributed to the decline in rates of respiratory complications among cases.

In conclusion, a change in the rates of respiratory complications and diarrhoea among cases occurred after 1979 in Gweru. It is suggested that the increase in vaccination coverage in 1979-89 and the shift in age at infection to older age groups in the same period may have brought about this change through selective suppression of occurrence of respiratory complications among measles cases

ACKNOWLEDGMENTS

This chapter is a revised version of an original paper published in the Journal of Tropical Pediatrics (Marufu T, Siziya S. Secular changes in rates of respiratory complications and diarrhoea among measles cases. J Trop Ped 1998; 44: 347-50) and the authors have obtained the permission from Journal of Tropical Pediatrics to use this material.

REFERENCES

[1] Makowiwitz LE, Orenstein WA. Measles vaccines. Pediatr Clin North Am 1990; 37: 603-25.

[19] Foster SO, McFarland DA, John AM. Measles. In: Jamison DT, Mosley WH, Measham AR, Bobadilla JL, eds. Disease control priorities in developing countries. New York: Oxford University Press, 1993: 161–87.

[20] Division of Diarrhoeal and Acute Respiratory Disease Control. Global programme for vaccines and immunization and expanded programme on immunization. Clinical research on treatment of measles: Report of a meeting. Banjul, Gambia. 3-5 November, 1993. Geneva: WHO/ CDR/95.15, WHO/EPI/GEN/95.07, 1993.

[21] Cutts FT. The immunological basis for immunization No. 7: Measles expanded programme on immunization. Geneva:WHO/EPI/GEN/93.17, 1993.

[22] Rodrigues LC. EPI target diseases: measles, tetanus, polio, tuberculosis, pertussis and diphtheria. In: Feachem RG, Jamison DT, eds. Disease and mortality in Sub-Saharan Africa. Oxford: Oxford University Press, 1991: 173-89.

[23] Kambarami RA, Nathoo KJ, Nkrumah FK, Pirie DJ. Measles epidemic in Harare, Zimbabwe despite high measles immunization coverage rates. Bull World Health Organ 1991; 69: 213-9.

[24] Marufu T, Siziya S, Tshimanga M, Murugasampillay S, Mason E, Manyame B. Factors associated with measles complications in Gweru, Zimbabwe. East Afr Med J 2001; 78: 135-8.

[25] Global Programme for Vaccines and Immunization. Immunization policy. Expanded programme on immunization. Geneva: WHO/EPI/GEN/95.3, 1995.

[26] Expanded Programme on Immunization. Measles control in the 1990s: Plan of action for global measles control. Geneva: WHO/EPI/GEN/92.3, 1992.

[27] Cutts FT. Measles control in the 1990's: Principles for the next decade. Expanded programme on immunization. Geneva: WHO/EPI/GEN/90.2, 1990.

[28] Markowitz LE, Nieburg P. The burden of acute respiratory infection due to measles in developing countries and the potential impact of measles vaccine. Rev Infect Dis 1991; 13(Suppl 6): S555-61.

[29] Stanfield SK, Shepard DS. Acute respiratory infection. In: Jamison DT, Mosley WH, Measham AR, Bobadilla JL, eds. Disease control priorities in developing countries. Oxford: World Bank, Oxford University Press, 1993:67-90.

[30] Marufu T. The changing age ecology of measles and its implications on measles control. Cent Afr J Med 1992; 38: 208-14.

[31] Khoo A, Ho CK, Ong TK, Khairul A. Measles: An experience in Sandakan Hospital, Sabah, 1990. Singapore Med J 1994; 35: 595-8.

[32] Arya LS, Taana I, Tahiri C, Saidali A, Singh M. Spectrum of complications of measles in Afghanistan: a study of 784 cases. J Trop Med Hyg 1987; 90: 117-22.

[33] Marufu T, Murugasampillay S, Siziya S, Manyame B, Silape Z, Xaba E, et al. Is the protection afforded measles vaccinees the same in children of all age groups? Cent Afr J Med 1995; 41: 144-7.

[34] Samb B, Aaby P, Whittle H, Seek AM, Simondon F. Decline in measles case fatality ratio after the introduction of measles immunization in rural Senegal. Am J Epidemiol 1997; 145: 51-7

[35] Aaby P. Malnutrition and overcrowding/intensive exposure in severe measles infection: review of community studies. Rev Infect Dis 1988; 10: 478-91.

[36] Aaby P, Bukh J, Lisse IM, da Silva MC. Further community studies on the role of overcrowding and intensive exposure on measles mortality. Rev Infect Dis 1988; 10: 474-7.

In: Measles
Editors: T. Marufu, S. Siziya et al.
ISBN: 978-1-63485-559-4

Chapter 12

IMPACT OF MALNUTRITION AND MEASLES MORTALITY ON CHILDREN UNDER FIVE YEARS OF AGE

Tawanda Marufu[1,*], MB ChB, MSc,
Seter Siziya[2], BA (Ed), MSc, PhD
and Willard Tinago[1], BSc, MSc, PhD

[1]Department of Community Medicine, College of Health Sciences, University of Zimbabwe, Harare, Zimbabwe,
[2]Department of Clinical Sciences, Copperbelt University School of Medicine, Ndola, Zambia

A study was carried out to determine secular changes in all-cause mortality rates for children aged <5 years in 1960-1989 and their association with measles and malnutrition mortality rates in the same age group in the same period in city of Gweru, Zimbabwe. The study utilized under-fives mortality data from births and deaths registration office and measles and malnutrition surveillance data obtained from Gweru city's public health department. Data was analysed in SPSS version 20 for windows and linear regression analysis was used to determine whether measles and malnutrition mortality rates were independent predictors of all-cause underfives mortality rates. It was found that in 1960-1989 underfives mortality rates from all causes were 10.2-63.7/1000 live births

---

* Corresponding author: Tawanda Marufu, University of Zimbabwe College of Health Sciences, Box A 178, Avondale, Harare, Zimbabwe. E-mail: marufut@yahoo.com.

(median = 28.7, Q_1 = 16.2, Q_3 = 42.6) and these rates significantly and linearly declined in this period (χ^2 for linear trend = 165.74, $p < 0.001$). Measles mortality rates among underfives significantly and linearly declined (χ^2 for linear trend=812.49, $p < 0.001$) while malnutrition mortality rates in the same age group also significantly and linearly declined (χ^2 for linear trend = 2411.54, $p < 0.001$) in underfives in 1960-1989. Linear regression analysis indicated that malnutrition mortality rates (Regression Coefficient = 0.072, 95% CI [0.039, 0.104], $p < 0.001$) and measles mortality rates (Regression Coefficient = 0.029, 95% CI [0.006, 0.052], $p = 0.020$) were independent predictors of all-cause underfives mortality rates with an adjusted coefficient of determination of 70.5% with malnutrition mortality rates uniquely explaining 21% of the variance in all-cause underfives mortality rates, while measles mortality rates uniquely explained 7% of the variance in all-cause underfives mortality rates. It was concluded that decline in malnutrition and measles mortality rates among underfives significantly contributed to decline in all-cause underfives mortality rates in 1960-89 in Gweru city, Zimbabwe. On account of these findings, it is critical that efforts directed at controlling malnutrition and measles be intensified in areas and populations of similar settings.

INTRODUCTION

Malnutrition and measles are known to contribute significantly to all-cause underfives mortality and, consequently, their control would contribute substantially to reduction in all-cause under-five mortality (1-3). Underfives mortality attributed to undernutrition has been estimated at 53-55% (2, 4) and on account of this it has been concluded that efforts directed at reducing malnutrition should be a policy priority (1). Measles was estimated to cause 7% (5) and 1% (6) of under-five mortality in 1990 and 2008 respectively. Measles control through improved vaccination efforts is estimated to have reduced all-cause child mortality by 23% in the period 1990-2008 (3). On account of the importance of malnutrition and measles to child deaths, a retrospective study that examined secular changes in all-cause underfives mortality in the period 1960-89 in the city of Gweru in Zimbabwe also explored the relationship between these secular changes and mortality attributed to measles and malnutrition in children of the same age group in the same period. This paper reports on this study.

OUR STUDY

Data on measles and malnutrition mortality, and mortality from all causes among underfives for the period 1960-1989 were reviewed. Secular trends in measles and malnutrition mortality rates, and rates of mortality from all causes among underfives were quantified. Association between all-cause underfives mortality rates, and measles and malnutrition mortality rates in the same age group were explored.

The following were the sources of data: (a) Data on deaths among underfives were obtained from the office of the registrar of births and deaths in Gweru, (b) Data on measles mortality among underfives was obtained from city of Gweru measles surveillance records. In Gweru measles cases are identified through a surveillance system that records cases and deaths that are reported from the city's health centres, community and the city's infectious disease hospital. Data on measles cases and deaths are entered on line lists that indicate date of identification of a case, age at infection, gender, vaccination status, presenting features, whether admitted into hospital or not, treatment and outcome of illness (alive or dead) and (c) Data on malnutrition mortality among underfives was obtained from Gweru city's nutrition surveillance system. In Gweru city public health department data on nutrition-associated mortality in underfives is collected as one of the items of the nutritional surveillance system. The data indicates date of death, age at death, gender and type of nutritional deficiency responsible for death.

The following were determined for each year in the period 1960-89: (a) All-cause mortality rates for underfives per 1000 live births, (b) Measles mortality rates per 100,000 population of children under five years of age and (c) Malnutrition mortality rates per 100,000 population of underfives. The data were entered into and analysed in SPSS version 20.0 for Windows. The Forward Stepwise Multiple Linear Regression method was used to determine whether measles and malnutrition mortality rates were independent predictors of all-cause mortality rates for underfives. The probability of the F test for the variable to enter the model was set at 5% and to remove was 6%.

FINDINGS

Measles and malnutrition mortality rates among underfives, and all-cause mortality rates for the same age group in the period 1960-1989 are indicated in Table 1 and Figure 1. In 1960-89 the all-cause mortality rates for underfives were 10.2-63.7 per 1000 live births (median: 28.7, Q_1 = 16.2, Q_3 = 42.6). These rates significantly and linearly declined in this period (χ^2 for linear trend = 165.74, $p < 0.001$).

Table 1. Measles and malnutrition mortality rates among underfives, and all-cause underfives mortality rates in Gweru city, Zimbabwe, 1960-1989

Year	All-cause underfives mortality rates /1000 live births	Measles mortality rates among underfives /100 000 population of underfives	Malnutrition mortality rates among underfives/100 000 population of underfives
1960	59.7	231.9	338.9
61	52.7	81.05	389
62	40.9	29.27	222.8
63	31.0	274.3	231
64	43.8	337.2	238.8
65	33.7	546.1	221.9
66	29.9	146.6	306.5
67	55.7	636.7	246.9
68	61.2	659.2	329.6
69	63.7	457.9	507.4
1970	31.7	305.5	70.5
71	41.1	190.1	22.4
72	36.9	96	117.3
73	47.0	163.2	50.9
74	43.1	136.8	136.8
75	27.4	28.1	74.9
76	18.5	36	18
77	18.8	43.4	43.4
78	12.4	25.1	25.1
79	25.9	80.7	64.6
1980	21.5	31.2	124.8
81	17.4	15.1	45.3
82	14.4	21.9	36.5
83	15.8	75.9	75.9
84	12.9	19.6	6.5
85	26.6	18.6	30.9
86	13.4	0	11.8
87	12.3	0	16.9
88	15.2	1	5.4
1989	10.2	0	15.5
Range			
Minimum	10.2	0	5.4
Maximum	63.7	659.2	507.4
Percentiles			
Q_1	16.2	22.7	25.6
Median	28.7	78.3	72.7
Q_3	42.6	221.45	228.9
Mean	31.2	156.3	134.2

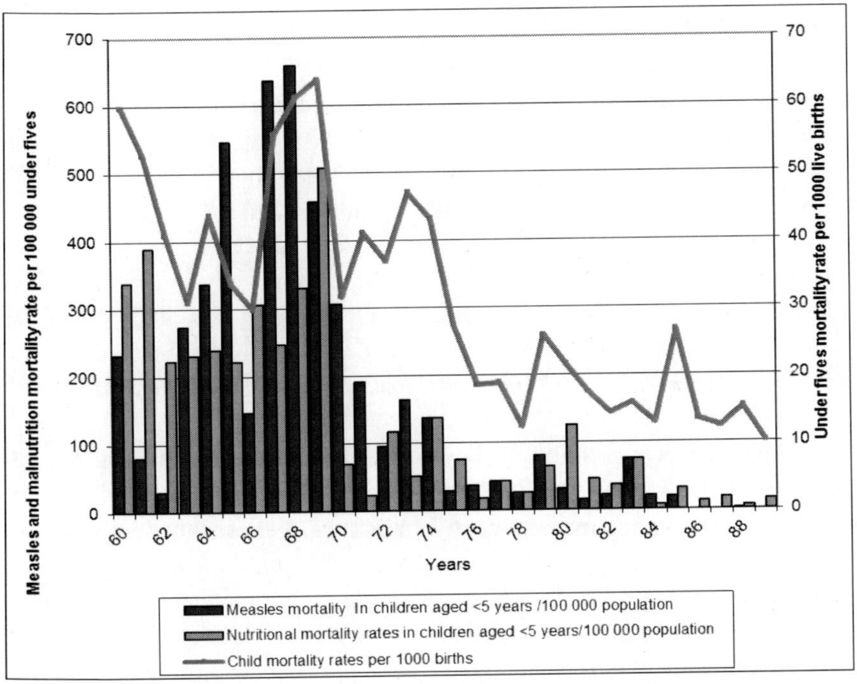

Figure 1. Measles and malnutrition mortality rates among underfives, and all-cause underfives mortality rates in Gweru city, Zimbabwe, 1960-1989.

In 1960-1989 measles mortality rates among underfives were 0 - 659.2 per 100,000 population (median: 78.3, $Q_1 = 22.7$, $Q_3 = 221.5$). These rates significantly and linearly declined in this period (χ^2 for linear trend = 812.49, $p < 0.001$). Malnutrition mortality rates among underfives in 1960-1989 were 5.4-507.4 per 100,000 population (median: 72.7, $Q_1 = 26.6$, $Q_3 = 228.9$). In this period these rates significantly and linearly declined (χ^2 for linear trend = 2411.54, $p < 0.001$).

Results from linear regression analysis indicated that malnutrition mortality rates among underfives (Regression Coefficient = 0.072, 95% CI [0.039-0.104], $p < 0.001$) and measles mortality rates in the same age group (Regression Coefficient = 0.029, 95% CI [0.006-0.052], $p = 0.020$) were independent predictors of all-cause underfives mortality rates with an adjusted coefficient of determination of 70.5% with malnutrition mortality rates uniquely explaining 21% of the variance in all-cause underfives mortality rates, while measles mortality rates uniquely explained 7% of the variance in all-cause underfives mortality rates.

DISCUSSION

This study found that all-cause mortality rates for underfives declined over the 30 year period 1960-89 and that this decline was associated with decline in malnutrition and measles mortality rates in this age group in the same period. Studies that have investigated secular trends of underfives mortality in developing countries have found that these mortality rates declined in the period 1960-89 (7-10) and thus findings of the current study concur with these studies. In Zimbabwe, like in the current study, underfives mortality declined in 1960-1990 (7, 8) but increased in the 1990s due to worsening economic conditions and the direct and indirect impact of the HIV/AIDS epidemic (8, 11).

In this study it was found that measles and malnutrition mortality rates among underfives declined in 1960-89. A study that examined secular trends in mortality attributed to measles in Gweru in 1967-89 found that both measles and malnutrition mortality rates had declined among under-fives in that period (12). From findings of the current study it would seem that decline in measles and malnutrition mortality rates observed in that study (12) are likely to have been a continuation of a trend that would have commenced in 1960 or before.

The current study found that in 1960-89 decline in malnutrition and measles mortality rates among underfives accounted for 70.5% of variation in all-cause underfives mortality rates. The implication of this finding is that in Gweru in this period malnutrition and measles may have been the conditions mostly associated with mortality among under-fives, probably meaning that oft mentioned factors such as neonatal disorders, pneumonia, diarrhoea and malaria that are said to be major causes of mortality among under-fives (8, 10, 13, 14) or factors such as socio-economic conditions that are known to have strong impact on underfives mortality in developing countries (15) would all seem to have contributed only 29.5% of the variation in all-cause underfives mortality. In 2000-03 major causes of underfives mortality in developing countries were said to be neonatal disorders, pneumonia and diarrhoea which were estimated to account for 73% of all underfives mortality while malaria, measles, HIV/AIDS, injuries and other causes accounted for the remaining 27% (14). Differences between major causes of mortality in Gweru in 1960-89 (as found in the current study) and estimates of major causes of underfives mortality indicated for 2000-03 for developing countries (14) seem to demonstrate that major causes of underfives mortality are period specific (as in time or era) (1) and area specific (as in geographical distribution) (13, 14).

The current study found that malnutrition mortality rates among underfives uniquely explained 21% of the variance in all-cause underfives mortality while measles mortality rates uniquely explained only 7% of the variance in all-cause mortality of the same age group. Malnutrition is an underlying cause of half of all deaths occurring among underfives in developing countries (13, 14, 16). Also, among underfives malnutrition is strongly associated with increased risk of mortality from diarrhoea, acute lower respiratory infections and pneumonia, malaria, and measles (13, 17). Studies indicated earlier (13, 14) have found that measles (compared to conditions such as pneumonia, diarrhoea, etc.) is associated with a small proportion of deaths among underfives in developing countries. The implication of this finding is, as found in the current study, that the effect of malnutrition mortality rates on all-cause underfives mortality rates would be much bigger compared to that of measles mortality rates on account of the fact that malnutrition is associated with a far greater proportion of underfives mortality compared to measles.

A major limitation of the current study was that variables that were examined were few. This is due to the fact that in1960-89 data relating to management and outcomes of factors associated with underfives mortality such as neonatal disorders, pneumonia, diarrhoea, malaria, etc. were for most part incomplete or inadequate. Equally, data that would have enabled measurement of impact of socio-economic conditions on underfives mortality were not available. In the absence of adequate data on these variables it was not possible to examine how they specifically contributed to decline in under-five mortality in 1960-89.

In conclusion, the decline in malnutrition and measles mortality rates among underfives significantly contributed to decline in all-cause underfives mortality rates in 1960-89 in Gweru city, Zimbabwe. On account of these findings, it is critical that efforts directed at controlling malnutrition and measles be intensified in areas and populations of similar settings.

ACKNOWLEDGMENTS

This chapter is a revised version of an original paper published in the European Journal of Preventive Medicine (Tawanda Marufu, Seter Siziya, Willard Tinago. Impact of malnutrition and measles mortality on underfives all-cause mortality in Gweru city, Zimbabwe, in 1960-89. Eur J Prev Med

2015; 3: 209-212) and the authors have obtained the permission from European Journal of Preventive Medicine to use this material.

References

[1] LE, de Onis M, Blossner M, Black RE. Undernutrition as an underlying cause of child deaths associated with diarrhoea, pneumonia, malaria, and measles. Am J Clin Nutr 2004; 80(1): 193-8.

[37] Pelletier DL, Frongillo EA Jr, Habicht JP. Epidemiologic evidence for a potentiating effect of malnutrition on child mortality. Am J Public Health 1993; 83(8): 1130-3.

[38] van den Ent MM, Brown DW, Hoekstra EJ, Christie A, Cochi SL. Measles mortality reduction contributes substantially to reduction of all-cause mortality among children less than five years of age, 1990-2008. J Infect Dis 2011; 204(Suppl 1): S18-23.

[39] Pelletier DL, Frongillo EA, Jr., Schroeder DG, Habicht JP. The effects of malnutrition on child mortality in developing countries Bull World Health Organ 1995; 73(4): 443-8.

[40] Lopez AD, Begg S, Bos E. Demographic and epidemiological characteristics of major regions, 1990-2001. In: Lopez AD, Mathers CD, Ezzati M, Jamison DT, Murray CJL, eds. Global burden of disease and risk factors. Washington, DC: World Bank, 2006.

[41] Black RE, Cousens S, Johnson HL, Lawn JE, Rudan I, Bassani DG, et al. Global, regional, and national causes of child mortality in 2008: a systematic analysis. Lancet 2010; 375(9730): 1969-87.

[42] Hill K, Pande R, Mahy M, Jones G. Trends in child mortality in the developing world: 1960-1996. New York: UNICEF, 1999.

[43] Hill K, Amouzou A. Trends in child mortality, 1960 to 2000. In: Jamison DT, Feachem RG, Makgoba MW, Bos ER, Baingana FK, Hofman KJ, Rogo KO, eds. Disease and mortality in sub-Saharan Africa. 2nd ed. Washington, DC: World Bank, 2006.

[44] Hill K, Pande R, Mahy M, Jones G. Trends in under-five mortality 1960-1990: estimates for 84 developing countries. Washington, DC: World Bank, 1994.

[45] Roll Back Malaria, UNICEF and World Health Organisation. World malaria report 2005: URL: http://www.rollbackmalaria.org/files/files/resources/WMReport_lr.pdf

[46] Central Statistical Office [Zimbabwe] and Macro International Inc. Zimbabwe demographic and health survey 1999. Calverton, MD: Macro International, 2002.

[47] Marufu T, Siziya S, Mudambo KS. Factors associated with secular trends in mortality attributed to measles in Gweru, Zimbabwe, in 1967-89. J Trop Pediatr 2008; 54(2): 114-9.

[48] Black RE, Morris SS, Bryce J. Where and why are 10 million children dying every year? Lancet 2003; 361(9376): 2226-34.

[49] Bryce J, Boschi-Pinto C, Shibuya K, Black RE. WHO estimates of the causes of death in children. Lancet 2005; 365(9465): 1147-52.

[50] Amouzou A, Hill K. Child mortality and socio-economic status in sub-Saharan Africa. Etude De La Population Africaine 2004; 19: 1-11

[51] Rice AL, Sacco L, Hyder A, Black RE. Malnutrition as an underlying cause of childhood deaths associated with infectious diseases in developing countries. Bull World Health Organ 2000; 78(10): 1207-21.

[52] Schroeder DG, Brown KH. Nutritional status as a predictor of child survival: summarizing the association and quantifying its global impact. Bull World Health Organ 1994; 72(4): 569-79.

Section four: Acknowledgments

In: Measles
Editors: T. Marufu, S. Siziya et al.
ISBN: 978-1-63485-559-4

Chapter 13

About the Editors

Tawanda Marufu, MB ChB, MSc was born in rural Chivi District in Zimbabwe. He is currently employed with the University of Zimbabwe College of Health Sciences in Harare, Zimbabwe, as a lecturer in the Department of Community Medicine. His work experience has included Director of Medical Services for the City of Gweru urban district in Zimbabwe, training consultant for the Rockefeller Foundation responsible for the development of MPH programme at the University of Zimbabwe (Rockefeller Foundation Public Health Schools without walls project), lecturer at the University of Zimbabwe Medical School, consultant medical officer for the WHO Polio Eradication Initative (in Nigeria, Ethiopia and Somalia), lecturer at the JMU Centre for Public Health (Liverpool, United Kingdom), and WHO Regional Medical Officer responsible for the Male Circumcision for HIV Prevention Programme for Eastern and Southern Africa (ESA). His research interests include epidemiology and control of diseases that are prevented through immunization, epidemiology and control of sexually transmitted infections/diseases (including HIV/AIDS) and epidemiology and control of non communicable diseases. He is a registered medical practioner, public health specialist and a Fellow of Royal Institute of Public Health (UK). E-mail: marufut@yahoo.com

Seter Siziya, BA(Ed), MSc, PhD, born in Lusaka, Zambia, is a professor of medical biostatistics with the Copperbelt University in the School of Medicine, Ndola Central Hospital in Zambia. He was recognized as one of the Hot 100 authors worldwide for the BioMedCentral Journals in 2007; awarded a certificate of achievement by the Copperbelt University for outstanding achievement in research at the Copperbelt University School of Medicine in 2012; Received a Vice-Chancellor's award for excellence for the years in 2013 at the Copperbelt University; and received a meritorious award for excellence in research and academic development from the Zambia Medical Association in 2013. He previously worked for the Tropical Diseases Research Centre, Ndola, Zambia; University of Zimbabwe and the University of Zambia. He has been teaching biostatistics, epidemiology and research methods to both undergraduate and postgraduate students in the universities he has worked in. He has been a reviewer, editorial member and associate editor for international journals. He has published numerous papers on tobacco smoking, HIV, Integrated management of childhood illnesses, immunization, measles, non-communicable diseases, suicide, bullying, alcohol and occupational health. He is a member of the Health Professions Council of Zambia and chairs its Education committee. E-mail: ssiziya@gmail.com

Mazyanga L Mazaba, BSc, MSc, born in Lusaka, Zambia, graduated from the University of Zambia, School of Medicine. She specialises in the areas of virology and public health (vaccines and preventable diseases). She is currently a National Professional Officer-laboratory scientist and data manager with the World Health Organization under the Expanded Program on Immunisation (EPI), particularly, polio, measles, rubella, influenza, rota virus and yellow fever surveillance and involved in laboratory diagnosis and training laboratory and surveillance personnel in sample collection and management. She has vast experience in immunology, virology, various diagnostic methods, data management, outbreak investigations and field epidemiology. She has published in a variety of peer reviewed journals and presented papers at international and national conferences in the field of virology and epidemiology. She is now working in the field of epidemiology as she pursues a DSc in epidemiology. E-mail: liwewema@who.int

Joav Merrick, MD, MMedSci, DMSc, born and educated in Denmark is professor of pediatrics, child health and human development, Division of Pediatrics, Hadassah Hebrew University Medical Center, Mt Scopus Campus, Jerusalem, Israel and Kentucky Children's Hospital, University of Kentucky, Lexington, Kentucky United States and professor of public health at the Center for Healthy Development, School of Public Health, Georgia State University, Atlanta, United States, the medical director of the Health Services, Division for Intellectual and Developmental Disabilities,

Ministry of Social Affairs and Social Services, Jerusalem, the founder and director of the National Institute of Child Health and Human Development in Israel. Numerous publications in the field of pediatrics, child health and human development, rehabilitation, intellectual disability, disability, health, welfare, abuse, advocacy, quality of life and prevention. Received the Peter Sabroe Child Award for outstanding work on behalf of Danish Children in 1985 and the International LEGO-Prize ("The Children's Nobel Prize") for an extraordinary contribution towards improvement in child welfare and well-being in 1987. E-mail: jmerrick@zahav.net.il

In: Measles
Editors: T. Marufu, S. Siziya et al.
ISBN: 978-1-63485-559-4

Chapter 14

About the College of Health Sciences at the University of Zimbabwe

The vision of the College of Health Sciences at the University of Zimbabwe is to be a referenced teaching, training, research and international leader in Africa and beyond in evidence based training, innovative student learning and health care delivery. The mission of the College is to provide an enabling environment for evidence based high quality, community oriented and community driven training and learning for health care professionals and for the college to be a clinical and research centre of excellence and a source of high quality health consultancy services.

History

The College of Health Sciences, formerly the Medical School, was established in 1963 under the auspices of the University of Birmingham as a joint initiative of the University College of Rhodesia and Nyasaland and University of Birmingham Medical School, United Kingdom. This was after the then Rhodesian Government realized the need for locally trained medical doctors. After wide consultations by the then government, the University of Birmingham in 1960 agreed to sponsor the proposed Medical School. In 1963, the first 26 students were enrolled for the Bachelor of Medicine and Bachelor of Surgery Degrees (MB ChB) at the University College of Rhodesia and Nyasaland. At the time the medical school was named after a former prime minister of Southern Rhodesia, Federation of Rhodesia and Nyasaland, Sir Godfrey Huggins and was therefore called Godfrey Huggins School of Medicine. The College of Health Sciences has undergone significant growth and expansion since inception in 1963. In the year 2000 it became the College of Health Sciences (CHS) and it ceased to be one of the faculties of the University of Zimbabwe. Currently the College has twenty-two teaching departments, one institute and one school.

Curriculum model

The College of Health Sciences utilizes an integrated and community oriented curriculum model across the years of training. It is migrating towards a competence based curriculum model where teaching and learning is geared towards the imparting and acquiring of specific competences under identified core competence domains at every level of training. The competence based curriculum model is an innovative approach to health care training and assists in developing wholesome healthcare practitioners. The community based curriculum components ensure culturally sensitive and contextually relevant health care practitioners upon completion of training.

Research activities

The college places great value on innovative and relevant high impact research. Research is central to our mandate with the overall aim of providing ethical and evidence based health care. To spearhead research and its management, the college established a Research Support Centre which offers research support services to staff and students. The College always seeks to enhance its grant acquisition capacity since health sciences research has become increasingly grant based. It has previously received and continues to receive and participate in collaborative grant based research including: the University of Zimbabwe–University of California San Francisco (UZ-UCSF) Collaborative Research and the Development of Anti-Retroviral Therapy (DART). As part of its research capacity building efforts, the College has also received prestigious research grants like, the Southern African Consortium for Research Excellence (SACORE) and the Medical Education Partnership

Initiative (MEPI) research grants and European and Developing Countries Clinical Trials Partnership (EDTCP).

Our Institute of Continuing Health Education holds an Annual Medical Research Day where health professionals showcase their research findings.

Linkages and partnerships

The College values linkages and partnerships to enhance teaching, learning and research. Through linkages and partnerships with health care training and research institutions across the globe, the College has participated and continues to participate in collaborative capacity building and operational research activities.Some of the linkages include; the University of Zimbabwe–University of California San Francisco (UZ-UCSF) Collaborative Research and the Development of Anti-Retroviral Therapy (DART). The linkages and partnerships have seen the College recently receiving research and capacity building grants like; the African Mental Health Initiative (AMARI), Promoting Excellence in Research and Faculty Training (PERFECT).

The College also has various memoranda of agreement and understanding with health care training institutions across the globe. These agreements facilitate staff and student exchange, among a host of other capacity building activities involved. Linkages and partnerships enable the College to benchmark its teaching, learning and research activities along international best practices. They also broadly strengthen the south-south and south-north cooperation.

Consultancy

The College leverages on its broad expertise base to offer high level consultancy services to various health care organisations locally, regionally and internationally. Various departments and individual members in the College are renowned focal points for consultancy services and offer technical assistance to the Ministry of Health and Child Care, Non-Governmental Organisations and international healthcare policy organisations.

Targets

The College of Health Sciences targets to become a centre of excellence in health care training and research. It targets to expand postgraduate training towards subspecialty training. This will consequently improve teaching, research and the quality of clinical service to the health seeking population of Zimbabwe. The College also targets to increase its grant acquisition capacity by training staff on grant writing and grant management skills. This will result in increased research activity and publication profiles for its members. In the long term, the College targets to establish a University Teaching Hospital wholly under its management.

Contacts

Dean, Professor Midion M Chidzonga
University of Zimbabwe College of Health Sciences
POBox A178, Avondale, Harare, Zimbabwe
E-mails: chsmainoffice@gmail.com, mtmchidzonga@yahoo.com

Lecturer, Dr Tawanda Marufu
Department of Community Medicine
University College of Health Sciences
POBox A 178, Avondale, Harare, Zimbabwe
E-mail: marufut@yahoo.com

In: Measles
Editors: T. Marufu, S. Siziya et al.
ISBN: 978-1-63485-559-4

Chapter 15

About the School of Medicine, Copperbelt University in Ndola, Zambia

The Copperbelt University School of Medicine (CBU SOM) was approved by the Senate of the Copperbelt University and inaugurated by the President of the republic of Zambia in June 2011 and the Zambia Health Professions Council approved the commencement of training in Dentistry and Medicine. The school admitted its inaugural class on the 14th November 2011. The school has three departments: Basic sciences, Clinical sciences (in which Public Health unit is housed) and Dental sciences. Copperbelt University School of Medicine is the second public Medical School in Zambia. It is the first Dental School in Zambia offering the Bachelors in Dental Surgery (BDS).

Mission

On establishment, the mission of the CBU SOM was to produce medical doctors and dentists who understand the health care context of the Zambian community, who will be able to convert their knowledge into solutions that will impact the care of the sick in Zambia. New programs have since been introduced including Bachelor of Science degree in clinical medicine, Master of Medicine in surgery, urology and obstetrics and gynaecology; Master of Science and Doctor of Science degrees by dissertation. Degrees by dissertation will produce senior and expert medical scientists who would manage academic research units and academic research departments or institutions within the university system or other similar institutions. This school's mission stems from the Copperbelt University mission which is "To contribute to the development and sustenance of the well-being of the people of Zambia and the world through the provision of flexible, innovative, entrepreneurial, inclusive programmes of teaching, learning, research and service ". In view of the new programs that have been introduced, the school's mission would need to be recast to take into consideration these new programs.

Curriculum model

The curriculum model is innovative. It is a modern approach to curriculum design which is open and integrative. It provides for vertical integration between the basic sciences and dental/medical practice, as well as horizontal integration of the basic sciences to each other. The curriculum allows for early exposure to dental/medical practice and continuous teaching in basic sciences throughout the programs. The curriculum uses a combination of delivery of curriculum of student centered and systems based learning to achieve a learning mix that produces the best in the student. Community based training is an integral part of the curriculum that runs throughout the programs and anchors the training within the context of the community. The model is open by breaking the subject specific system of training in favour of learning by concept system. During the MSc and DSc programs, students are exposed to non-examinable modules in medical sciences, research methods, leadership and administration.

Research activities

The school has a research coordinator. There are three research groups, namely: basic sciences, clinical sciences and public health. Under basic sciences, the study areas are tuberculosis, nutrition, anatomy organs and weight, and schistosomiasis; in the clinical group the topics are circumcision, and under public health group, the study areas are maternal and child health, non-communicable diseases, substance abuse among adolescents, integrated management of childhood diseases, infectious diseases and health systems.

Linkages and partnerships

The CBU SOM collaborates with local research institutions that include the Tropical Diseases Research Centre and the School of Medicine of the University of Zambia. Internationally, it is part of two consortia, the Consortium of New Medical Schools (CONSAMS) that include the University of Namibia, University of Botswana, University of Lurio in Mozambique, University of Lesotho, Oulu University in Finland and the University of Vanderbilt in the USA. The other consortium is the Medical Education Initiative which consists of 13 Universities in Africa and is funded under a National Health Institute program of the USA government. The School recently commenced an international collaboration with the University of Tel Aviv in Israel, spearheaded mainly through teaching of the new MPH program to commence in 2016. The school is open to creating more linkages and partnerships worldwide to be part of the research and teaching communities in solving local and international health problems.

Consultancy

The school has varied expertise reflected in the teaching programs. CBU SOM provides consultancies in line with and outside the research activities of the school. The School provides consultancies to several institutions including the Ministry of Health, the World Health Organization (National and International Office) and The National Science Research Council.

Targets

Building from the Copperbelt University vision of "To be an institution in which scholarship flourishes in an environment characterised by world class infrastructure and collaborative relations and supported by an accountable, transparent and efficient University governance system ", the school hopes to produce sufficient doctors and dentist to meet the WHO recommendation of 1 doctor per 5000 population, 1:10,000 and one specialist per 10,000 populations, 1:300,000 respectively. Through this to improve the health indices in Zambia to the level obtaining in developed countries. Through research collaboration with other institutions (locally and internationally), the school will become a centre of excellence in research.

Contacts

Mrs. Helen Mwenya Mukumba
Registrar, Copperbelt University, Jambo Drive, Riverside
POBox 21692, Kitwe, Zambia
E-mail: registrar@cbu.ac.zm

Professor Seter Siziya
Clinical Sciences Department, School of Medicine
POBox 71191, Ndola, Zambia
E-mail: ssiziya@gmail.com

In: Measles
Editors: T. Marufu, S. Siziya et al.
ISBN: 978-1-63485-559-4

Chapter 16

About the National Institute of Child Health and Human Development in Israel

The National Institute of Child Health and Human Development (NICHD) in Israel was established in 1998 as a virtual institute under the auspices of the Medical Director, Ministry of Social Affairs and Social Services in order to function as the research arm for the Office of the Medical Director. In 1998 the National Council for Child Health and Pediatrics, Ministry of Health and in 1999 the Director General and Deputy Director General of the Ministry of Health endorsed the establishment of the NICHD.

Mission

The mission of a National Institute for Child Health and Human Development in Israel is to provide an academic focal point for the scholarly interdisciplinary study of child life, health, public health, welfare, disability, rehabilitation, intellectual disability and related aspects of human development. This mission includes research, teaching, clinical work, information and public service activities in the field of child health and human development.

Service and academic activities

Over the years many activities became focused in the south of Israel due to collaboration with various professionals at the Faculty of Health Sciences (FOHS) at the Ben Gurion University of the Negev (BGU). Since 2000 an affiliation with the Zusman Child Development Center at the Pediatric Division of Soroka University Medical Center has resulted in collaboration around the establishment of the Down Syndrome Clinic at that center. In 2002 a full course on "Disability" was established at the Recanati School for Allied Professions in the Community, FOHS, BGU and in 2005 collaboration was started with the Primary Care Unit of the faculty and disability became part of the master of public health course on "Children and society". In the academic year 2005-2006 a one semester course on "Aging with disability" was started as part of the master of science program in gerontology in our collaboration with the Center for Multidisciplinary Research in Aging. In 2010 collaborations with the Division of Pediatrics, Hadassah Hebrew University Medical Center, Jerusalem, Israel around the National Down Syndrome Center and teaching students and residents about intellectual and developmental disabilities as part of their training at this campus.

Research activities

The affiliated staff have over the years published work from projects and research activities in this national and international collaboration. In the year 2000 the International Journal of Adolescent Medicine and Health and in 2005 the International Journal on Disability and Human Development of De Gruyter Publishing House (Berlin and New York) were affiliated with the National Institute of Child Health and Human Development. From 2008 also the International Journal of Child Health and Human Development (Nova Science, New York), the International Journal of Child and Adolescent Health (Nova Science) and the Journal of Pain Management (Nova Science) affiliated and from 2009 the International Public Health Journal (Nova Science) and Journal of Alternative Medicine Research (Nova Science). All peer-reviewed international journals.

National collaborations

Nationally the NICHD works in collaboration with the Faculty of Health Sciences, Ben Gurion University of the Negev; Department of Physical Therapy, Sackler School of Medicine, Tel Aviv University; Autism Center, Assaf HaRofeh Medical Center; National Rett and PKU Centers at Chaim Sheba Medical Center, Tel HaShomer; Department of Physiotherapy, Haifa University; Department of Education, Bar Ilan University, Ramat Gan, Faculty of Social Sciences and Health Sciences; College of Judea and Samaria in Ariel and in 2011 affiliation with Center for Pediatric Chronic Diseases and National Center for Down Syndrome, Department of Pediatrics, Hadassah Hebrew University Medical Center, Mount Scopus Campus, Jerusalem.

International collaborations

Internationally with the Department of Disability and Human Development, College of Applied Health Sciences, University of Illinois at Chicago; Strong Center for Developmental Disabilities, Golisano Children's Hospital at Strong, University of Rochester School of Medicine and Dentistry, New York; Centre on Intellectual Disabilities, University of Albany, New York; Centre for Chronic Disease Prevention and Control, Health Canada, Ottawa; Chandler Medical Center and Children's Hospital, Kentucky Children's Hospital, Section of Adolescent Medicine, University of Kentucky, Lexington; Chronic Disease Prevention and Control Research Center, Baylor College of Medicine, Houston, Texas; Division of Neuroscience, Department of Psychiatry, Columbia University, New York; Institute for the Study of Disadvantage and Disability, Atlanta; Center for Autism and Related Disorders, Department Psychiatry, Children's Hospital Boston, Boston; Department of Pediatric and Adolescent Medicine, Western Michigan University Homer Stryker MD School of Medicine, Kalamazoo, Michigan, United States; Department of Paediatrics, Child Health and Adolescent Medicine, Children's Hospital at Westmead, Westmead, Australia; International Centre for the Study of Occupational and Mental Health, Düsseldorf, Germany; Centre for Advanced Studies in Nursing, Department of General Practice and Primary Care, University of Aberdeen, Aberdeen, United Kingdom; Quality of Life Research Center, Copenhagen, Denmark; Nordic School of Public Health, Gottenburg, Sweden, Scandinavian Institute of Quality of Working Life, Oslo, Norway;

The Department of Applied Social Sciences (APSS) of The Hong Kong Polytechnic University Hong Kong.

Targets

Our focus is on research, international collaborations, clinical work, teaching and policy in health, disability and human development and to establish the NICHD as a permanent institute in Israel in order to conduct model research and together with the four university schools of public health/medicine in Israel establish a national master and doctoral program in disability and human development at the institute to secure the next generation of professionals working in this often non-prestigious/low-status field of work.

Contact

Joav Merrick, MD, MMedSci, DMSc
Professor of Pediatrics, Child Health and Human Development
Medical Director, Health Services, Division for Intellectual and Developmental Disabilities, Ministry of Social Affairs and Social Services, POB 1260, IL-91012 Jerusalem, Israel.
E-mail: jmerrick@zahav.net.il

In: Measles
Editors: T. Marufu, S. Siziya et al.
ISBN: 978-1-63485-559-4

Chapter 17

About the Book Series "Public Health: Practices, Methods and Policies"

Public health is a book series with publications from a multidisciplinary group of researchers, practitioners and clinicians for an international professional forum interested in the broad spectrum of public health issues. Books already published:

- Rubin IL, Merrick J, eds. Environment and public health: Environmental health, law and international perspectives. New York: Nova Science, 2014.
- Shek DTL, Siu AMH, Merrick J, eds. Tomorrow's leaders: Service leadership and holistic development in Chinese university students. New York: Nova Science, 2015.
- Siziya S, Mazaba ML, Merrick J, eds. Arbovirus: Public health experience from Zambia. New York: Nova Science, 2015.
- Obeng C, Obeng SG, Merrick J, eds. Health issues in diverse cultures. New York: Nova Science, 2015.
- Friedman BD, Merrick J, eds. Public health, social work and health inequalities. New York: Nova Science, 2015.
- Rubin IL, Merrick J, eds. Environmental health disparities: Costs and benefits of breaking the cycle. New York: Nova Science, 2016.
- *Mazaba ML, Siziya S, Merrick J, eds. Smoking and adolescence: International public health experiences. New York: Nova Science, 2016.*
- Merrick J, ed. Public health: Some international perspectives. New York: Nova Science, 2016.

- Greydanus DE, Merrick J. Medical history: Some perspectives. New York: Nova Science, 2016.
- Rubin IL, Merrick J, eds. Public health: International aspects on environment and health. New York: Nova Science, 2016.
- Shek DTL, Ma C, Lin L, Merrick J, eds. Education in Hong Kong: Service leadership for university students. New York: Nova Science, 2016.
- Shek DTL, Siu AMH, Leung H, Merrick J, eds. Higher Education in Hong Kong: Nurturing Students to be Caring Service Leaders. New York: Nova Science, 2016.

Contact

Professor Joav Merrick, MD, MMedSci, DMSc
Medical Director, Health Services
Division for Intellectual and Developmental Disabilities
Ministry of Social Affairs and Social Services
POBox 1260, IL-91012 Jerusalem, Israel
E-mail: jmerrick@zahav.net.il

SECTION FIVE: INDEX

INDEX

A

active measles surveillance, 15, 29, 57, 65, 74
adolescents, 134
adults, 21, 77, 100
advocacy, 127
Afghanistan, 100, 103, 109, 112
Africa, 4, 7, 8, 10, 14, 24, 34, 40, 43, 84, 93, 102, 103, 111, 125, 129, 135
age, 4, 5, 6, 7, 8, 9, 13, 14, 15, 16, 17, 18, 19, 20, 21, 23, 27, 28, 29, 30, 31, 32, 33, 34, 35, 36, 37, 38, 39, 40, 41, 42, 43, 44, 46, 47, 48, 51, 55, 56, 57, 58, 59, 60, 61, 62, 63, 64, 65, 66, 67, 68, 69, 70, 71, 72, 73, 74, 75, 76, 77, 78, 84, 85, 86, 87, 91, 95, 96, 97, 98, 99, 100, 101, 102, 106, 108, 109, 110, 112, 113, 114, 115, 117, 118, 119, 120
age at infection, 14, 15, 21, 23, 28, 29, 33, 36, 42, 57, 61, 65, 74, 77, 84, 95, 96, 97, 100, 102, 106, 108, 109, 110, 115
all-cause under-five mortality, 114
anatomy, 134
ANOVA, 105, 106
antibody, 52
assessment, 43, 46, 47, 50
attack rate, 48, 66

B

Bangladesh, 93, 102, 104
base, 131
benefits, 92, 141
birth rate, 20
births, 113, 115, 116
bivariate analysis, 97, 101
blood, 52
Botswana, 40, 135
bronchitis, 40
bronchopneumonia, 100, 109
bullying, 126
Burundi, 41, 50, 68, 69, 70, 77, 79

C

campaigns, 14, 36, 42
capacity building, 130, 131
Caribbean, 77
Caribbean countries, 77
case based measles surveillance, 7
case fatality rates, 36, 40, 41, 83, 84, 85, 86, 87, 88, 89, 90, 91, 92, 100, 101, 102, 106
cases aged >60 months, 56, 57
CDC, 8, 34, 52
Census, 24, 96
certificate, 125
challenges, 9, 25

change in age at infection, 33, 100, 110
Chicago, 139
child mortality, 8, 24, 114, 120
childhood, 22, 32, 101, 104, 121, 126, 134
children, 4, 5, 6, 7, 8, 9, 14, 15, 21, 22, 23, 28, 32, 34, 36, 37, 38, 40, 41, 42, 44, 46, 47, 48, 49, 50, 52, 55, 56, 57, 58, 60, 61, 62, 63, 64, 65, 66, 67, 68, 69, 71, 72, 73, 74, 75, 77, 78, 84, 85, 86, 87, 88, 89, 90, 91, 92, 100, 101, 102, 104, 109, 112, 113, 114, 115, 120
circumcision, 134
cities, 40, 72, 74, 75, 76, 77, 78
classes, 73
collaboration, 135, 138, 139
communities, 5, 15, 21, 22, 29, 32, 36, 42, 57, 65, 74, 92, 135
community, 6, 7, 21, 28, 29, 33, 36, 42, 43, 44, 47, 48, 56, 61, 65, 66, 69, 71, 73, 77, 84, 93, 96, 103, 104, 106, 110, 112, 115, 129, 130, 133, 134
complicated measles, 4, 81, 83, 84, 92
Complicated measles cases, 84
complications, 22, 24, 37, 39, 40, 44, 84, 85, 86, 87, 89, 90, 91, 92, 95, 96, 97, 98, 99, 100, 101, 102, 103, 105, 106, 107, 108, 109, 110, 111, 112
complications among the vaccinated cases, 101
conference, 7
confounding variables, 97
Congo, 50, 68
cooperation, 131
cross sectional study, 95
cross-sectional study, 96
croup, 40, 100, 106, 107, 108, 109, 110
curriculum, 130, 134
cycles, 51

D

DART, 130, 131
deaths, 8, 15, 29, 36, 37, 48, 51, 66, 84, 85, 91, 96, 97, 98, 99, 100, 101, 102, 106, 108, 110, 113, 114, 115, 119, 120, 121
deaths among complicated cases, 97
deficiency, 85, 115
dehydration, 100, 110
Denmark, 126, 139
dentist, 135
Department of Education, 139
dependent variable, 15
developed countries, 32, 108, 135
developing countries, 4, 5, 8, 9, 21, 22, 25, 28, 32, 33, 34, 36, 40, 42, 43, 44, 50, 60, 61, 62, 68, 69, 70, 77, 79, 91, 93, 100, 103, 104, 108, 111, 112, 118, 119, 120, 121
diarrhea, 8, 40, 100, 107, 110
diarrhoea, 4, 86, 87, 89, 90, 91, 93, 95, 97, 98, 99, 100, 101, 102, 105, 106, 107, 108, 109, 110, 111, 118, 119, 120
direct measure, 91
disability, 28, 34, 127, 137, 138, 140
diseases, 8, 15, 21, 24, 26, 29, 34, 36, 51, 57, 65, 74, 92, 93, 103, 104, 111, 121, 125, 126, 134
distribution, 4, 15, 17, 41, 118
doctors, 129, 133, 135
draft, 62, 70, 79

E

ecology, 8, 51, 62, 70, 112
economic status, 121
editors, 125
elementary school, 38
encephalitis, 98, 100, 107, 108
enteritis, 109
environment, 20, 129, 135, 142
epidemic, 7, 9, 17, 20, 25, 34, 39, 40, 43, 44, 48, 50, 52, 61, 62, 70, 79, 100, 103, 110, 111, 118
epidemiology, 3, 10, 14, 24, 28, 34, 36, 125, 126

evidence, 7, 42, 50, 120, 129, 130
Expanded Programme on Immunization (EPI), 3, 9, 14, 25, 34, 43, 44, 51, 52, 56, 62, 68, 70, 79, 93, 97, 103, 104, 109, 111, 126
expertise, 131, 135
exposure, 85, 97, 103, 110, 112, 134
extraction, 23, 33

F

Finland, 135
force, 9, 27, 28, 29, 30, 31, 32, 33
force of infection, 9, 27, 28, 29, 30, 31, 32, 33
formula, 47, 48, 66

G

gastroenteritis, 100
gender, 36, 57, 65, 74, 84, 85, 95, 96, 97, 98, 99, 101, 102, 106, 115
Georgia, 3, 126
Germany, 139
gerontology, 138
governance, 135
grants, 130, 131
growth, 92, 130
growth rate, 92
Guinea, 44, 101, 104

H

health, 4, 5, 8, 9, 14, 15, 28, 29, 36, 37, 40, 46, 47, 48, 51, 56, 57, 64, 65, 66, 73, 84, 93, 95, 96, 106, 115, 120, 126, 129, 130, 131, 132, 133, 134, 135, 137, 140, 141, 142
health care, 36, 47, 65, 129, 130, 131, 132, 133
health care professionals, 129
health problems, 135
heterogeneity, 24
history, 6, 26, 38, 55, 57, 72, 73, 102, 142
HIV, 4, 50, 52, 118, 125, 126
HIV/AIDS, 4, 118, 125
Hong Kong, 140, 142
horizontal integration, 134
hospitalization, 36, 57, 65, 74
host, 131
House, 83, 138
human, 52, 126, 137, 140
human development, 126, 137, 140
human immunodeficiency virus, 52
hypothesis, 56, 64, 73

I

identification, 84, 96, 106, 115
image, 31
immunity, 21, 22, 23, 25, 26, 28, 32, 33, 34, 60, 77
immunization, 4, 5, 7, 9, 24, 25, 34, 43, 44, 52, 62, 69, 70, 79, 84, 91, 101, 103, 104, 111, 112, 125, 126
immunization policy, 5, 9, 34, 62, 70, 79, 104, 111
improvements, 91
incidence, 4, 7, 13, 15, 16, 17, 19, 20, 21, 22, 23, 37, 55, 56, 58, 59, 60, 61, 63, 65, 66, 67, 69, 72, 73, 75, 76, 77, 84, 85, 86, 87, 88, 89, 91, 92
index case, 109
India, 92, 93, 102
individuals, 61
industrialized countries, 50, 68
inequality, 34
infancy, 21, 61, 77
infants, 40
infection, 5, 9, 14, 15, 16, 21, 23, 24, 27, 28, 29, 30, 31, 32, 33, 34, 36, 41, 42, 44, 50, 52, 57, 61, 65, 68, 74, 77, 84, 92, 95, 96, 97, 100, 101, 102, 103, 104, 106, 108, 109, 110, 112, 115
infrastructure, 135

injuries, 4, 118
injury, vi
institutions, 47, 131, 134, 135
interference, 68
intervention, 6, 43, 56, 58, 63, 71, 73
IQR, 15
Israel, 3, 126, 135, 137, 138, 140, 142
issues, 141
Ivory Coast, 7

J

Japan, 51
Jordan, 9, 22, 25, 34, 40, 42, 44, 62, 77, 79

L

Latin America, 77
lead, 41, 56, 73, 109
leadership, 134, 141, 142
learning, 129, 130, 131, 134
living conditions, 6, 20, 74
Luo, 44, 104

M

magnitude, 16, 29
majority, 91
malaria, 4, 8, 118, 119, 120
Malaysia, 109
malnutrition, 4, 8, 40, 83, 89, 91, 92, 97, 98, 100, 103, 107, 108, 110, 112, 113, 114, 115, 116, 117, 118, 119, 120, 121
management, 4, 8, 44, 84, 91, 92, 119, 126, 130, 132, 134
mass, 6, 36, 55, 57, 58, 60, 61, 71, 73, 75, 78
mass measles vaccination campaign, 61
maternal antibodies, 5, 6, 32, 40, 46, 50, 51, 64, 68
matter, 22, 91
Measles, 1, 3, 4, 5, 6, 7, 8, 9, 10, 11, 13, 14, 15, 16, 17, 18, 19, 20, 21, 22, 23, 24, 25, 26, 27, 28, 29, 30, 32, 33, 34, 35, 36, 37, 38, 39, 40, 41, 42, 43, 44, 45, 46, 47, 48, 49, 50, 51, 52, 53, 55, 56, 57, 58, 59, 60, 61, 62, 63, 64, 65,66, 67, 68, 69, 70, 71, 72, 73, 74, 75, 76, 77, 78, 79, 81, 83, 84, 85, 86, 87, 88, 89, 90, 91, 92, 93, 95, 96, 97, 98, 99, 100, 101, 102, 103, 104, 105, 106, 107, 108, 109, 110, 111, 112, 113, 114, 115, 116, 117, 118, 119, 120, 126
Measles complications, 24, 40, 44, 95, 96, 97, 102, 106, 108, 111
Measles epidemics, 5, 7, 22, 35, 41, 48, 72, 75
measles incidence rates, 4, 7, 13, 15, 16, 17, 20, 21, 22, 23, 55, 56, 58, 59, 60, 61, 63, 65, 66, 67, 69, 72, 73, 75, 76, 77, 84, 85, 86, 87, 88, 89, 91
measles mortality, 4, 8, 10, 22, 24, 42, 83, 84, 93, 100, 102, 103, 110, 112, 113, 114, 115, 116, 117, 118, 119, 120
measles transmission rates, 28, 33
Measles vaccination, 4, 6, 7, 8, 9, 10, 13, 14, 15, 18, 20, 24, 25, 28, 29, 35, 36, 37, 44, 46, 47, 48, 49, 50, 51, 52, 55, 56, 57, 58, 60, 61, 62, 63, 64, 65, 68, 69, 70, 71, 72, 73, 74, 75, 78, 79, 84, 85, 89, 100, 101, 104
measles vaccine coverage rates, 5, 6, 7, 15, 16, 17, 18, 20, 21, 27, 28, 58, 61, 77, 88, 89, 90, 91
measles vaccinees, 9, 44, 46, 62, 112
measurement, 119
media, 108
median, 13, 17, 18, 29, 56, 59, 60, 67, 72, 75, 76, 83, 85, 87, 89, 107, 109, 114, 116, 117
medical, 92, 125, 126, 129, 133, 134
medical care, 92
medical science, 134
medicine, 133, 140
methodology, 29

migration, 20
mission, 129, 133, 137
modules, 134
morbidity, 28, 36, 38, 40, 51, 92, 101
mortality, 4, 8, 10, 14, 22, 23, 24, 28, 36, 37, 40, 42, 44, 81, 83, 84, 85, 86, 87, 89, 90, 91, 92, 93, 96, 99, 100, 101, 102, 103, 104, 110, 111, 112, 113, 114, 115, 116, 117, 118, 119, 120, 121
mortality rate, 36, 37, 40, 85, 86, 87, 90, 92, 99, 101, 110, 113, 115, 116, 117, 118, 119
Mozambique, 40, 43, 135
multiple dose measles vaccination project, 7, 74
multiple dose measles vaccination strategies, 53, 56, 73
multiple dose vaccination schedules, 7
multiple dose vaccination strategies, 7, 72
multivariate analysis, 104
mumps, 26, 34

N

Namibia, 135
next generation, 140
Nigeria, 125
Nobel Prize, 127
Norway, 139
nutrition, 92, 93, 115, 134
nutritional deficiencies, 85
nutritional status, 84, 85, 92

O

occupational health, 126
operations, 51
organs, 134
otitis media, 98, 100, 107, 108

P

participants, 97
peer review, 126
permission, 24, 33, 43, 51, 62, 69, 78, 92, 103, 111, 120
pertussis, 93, 103, 111
PKU, 139
playing, 46
PM, 24
pneumonia, 4, 8, 40, 100, 101, 106, 107, 108, 109, 110, 118, 119, 120
policy, 5, 7, 9, 21, 22, 34, 42, 62, 70, 79, 91, 104, 111, 114, 131, 140
policy issues, 5
polio, 93, 103, 111, 126
population, 6, 7, 13, 14, 15, 16, 17, 20, 22, 23, 29, 32, 35, 36, 38, 40, 41, 46, 47, 48, 49, 55, 56, 57, 59, 64, 65, 67, 72, 73, 75, 76, 84, 85, 86, 87, 88, 89, 96, 101, 106, 115, 116, 117, 132, 135
population group, 7
population growth, 20
President, 133
pre-vaccination period, 17, 28
prevention, 34, 127
principles, 6, 7, 44
probability, 85, 115
professionals, 131, 138, 140
project, 6, 7, 10, 56, 57, 58, 60, 64, 65, 66, 73, 74, 125
protection, 7, 9, 10, 34, 42, 44, 62, 63, 64, 66, 69, 79, 101, 102, 112
prototype, 9, 25, 34, 44, 62, 79
public health, 7, 21, 22, 113, 115, 125, 126, 134, 137, 138, 140, 141
public service, 137
PVC, 48

Q

quality of life, 127

quasi-experimental community intervention, 6, 56, 71, 73

R

rates of all complications among cases, 107
rates of mortality, 83, 85, 86, 87, 89, 90, 91, 92, 96, 101, 115
rates of mortality among complicated measles cases, 84, 89, 90, 91
recommendations, 9, 25, 93
regression, 13, 85, 97, 99, 101, 113, 117
regression analysis, 13, 85, 97, 99, 101, 113, 117
rehabilitation, 127, 137
requirements, 65
research institutions, 131, 135
researchers, 141
resources, 120
Respiratory complications, 85, 86, 87, 89, 90, 91, 95, 97, 98, 99, 100, 102, 105, 106, 107, 108, 109, 110, 111
response, 7, 24, 50, 102
Revaccination, 6, 7, 10, 36, 42, 55, 57, 58, 60, 61, 62, 63, 64, 65, 66, 67, 68, 69, 72, 73, 74, 77, 79
revaccination schedules., 10, 62, 64, 66, 69, 79
risk, 5, 7, 21, 42, 52, 64, 66, 67, 68, 69, 96, 100, 102, 104, 108, 119, 120
risk factors, 52, 104, 120
risk of serious measles complications, 100
root, 50
Routine vaccinations, 15, 29, 57, 73
rubella, 9, 25, 26, 34, 126
Rwanda, 100

S

schistosomiasis, 134
scholarship, 135
school, 5, 22, 35, 37, 38, 41, 42, 73, 129, 133, 134, 135, 140
Schwarz strain vaccine, 36, 56, 64
science, 138
secular changes in all-cause underfives mortality, 114
self-control, 73
Senate, 133
services, 43, 65, 129, 131
sex, 15, 29
sexually transmitted infections, 125
siblings, 22, 36, 41, 42
significance level, 13
signs, 47
simple linear regression, 16
Singapore, 112
single dose and multiple dose measles vaccination strategies, 9, 25, 71, 72
single vaccination, 7, 63, 64, 66, 67, 68, 69
society, 138
Somalia, 125
South Africa, 22, 41, 42, 77
spectrum of complications, 100, 103, 108, 112
spectrum of measles complications, 107
statistics, 15, 29
stomatitis, 98, 100, 107, 108
storage, 46
structure, 6, 74, 100
sub-Saharan Africa, 93, 120, 121
substance abuse, 134
suicide, 126
supplementary measles immunization, 4, 84
supplementary measles immunization activities, 4, 84
support services, 130
suppression, 106, 109, 111
surveillance, 6, 7, 13, 15, 21, 23, 27, 28, 29, 33, 35, 36, 37, 46, 47, 55, 57, 58, 63, 65, 66, 72, 74, 83, 84, 85, 95, 96, 97, 106, 113, 115, 126
survival, 91, 92, 121
susceptibility, 5, 21, 23, 31, 32
Sweden, 139
symptoms, 47

T

Tanzania, 50, 68
target, 15, 56, 69, 77, 93, 103, 111
target population, 15
technical assistance, 131
tetanus, 93, 103, 111
tobacco, 126
tobacco smoking, 126
tonsillitis, 40, 107
training, 125, 126, 129, 130, 131, 132, 133, 134, 138
transmission, 4, 5, 6, 7, 8, 9, 13, 14, 16, 20, 21, 22, 23, 24, 25, 26, 27, 28, 29, 31, 32, 33, 34, 35, 36, 39, 40, 42, 43, 46, 47, 51, 55, 56, 57, 60, 62, 69, 71, 73, 77, 78, 79
transmission patterns, 4, 6, 8, 9, 13, 14, 23, 24, 25, 28, 35, 36, 43, 55, 56, 62, 71, 73, 79
transmission patterns of measles, 14
treatment, 15, 29, 36, 44, 57, 65, 74, 84, 91, 93, 103, 111, 115
trends of underfives mortality, 118
trial, 92
tuberculosis, 93, 103, 111, 134

U

underfives mortality, 4, 113, 114, 115, 116, 117, 118, 119
undernutrition, 8, 101, 114, 120
United Kingdom, 125, 129, 139
United States, 3, 126, 139
universities, 126
unvaccinated cases, 35, 37, 38, 39, 41, 46, 47, 61, 66, 67, 78, 96, 98, 99, 101, 102, 108
urban, 13, 15, 20, 24, 43, 64, 125
urban areas, 20
urban population, 20
USA, 32, 135

V

vaccinated cases, 4, 14, 18, 41, 42, 48, 49, 50, 55, 56, 59, 74, 76, 98, 99, 101, 109
vaccination, 4, 5, 6, 7, 8, 10, 13, 14, 15, 16, 17, 18, 19, 20, 21, 22, 23, 24, 26, 27, 28, 29, 32, 33, 34, 35, 36, 37, 40, 41, 42, 46, 47, 48, 49, 50, 51, 52, 55, 56, 57, 58, 59, 60, 61, 63, 64, 65, 66, 67, 68, 69, 71, 73, 74, 75, 77, 78, 84, 89, 95, 96, 97, 98, 99, 100, 101, 102, 104, 106, 108, 109, 110, 114, 115
vaccination coverage rates, 15, 17, 18, 21, 28, 29, 33, 41, 60, 65, 74, 78, 100, 110
vaccination fail, 46, 48, 50, 51, 69
vaccination schedules, 64
vaccination status of cases, 15, 29, 48, 57, 66, 95, 97, 108
vaccination strategy, 71
vaccinations, 6, 15, 28, 47, 57, 65, 67, 73, 74, 84
vaccine, 4, 5, 6, 7, 9, 13, 14, 15, 16, 17, 18, 19, 20, 21, 22, 23, 25, 26, 27, 28, 29, 32, 33, 34, 36, 37, 40, 41, 42, 43, 45, 46, 47, 48, 49, 50, 51, 55, 56, 57, 58, 59, 60, 61, 62, 64, 65, 66, 67, 68, 69, 70, 71, 72, 73, 74, 75, 77, 78, 79, 88, 89, 90, 91, 101, 104, 112
vaccine coverage rates, 4, 5, 6, 14, 15, 16, 17, 18, 20, 21, 22, 23, 28, 29, 32, 33, 40, 41, 56, 58, 61, 72, 75, 89
vaccine efficacy, 5, 6, 7, 9, 40, 43, 46, 47, 48, 49, 50, 51, 61, 64, 66, 68, 70, 77
Vaccine efficacy studies, 5, 51, 64, 68
vaccine failures, 4, 5, 6, 7, 14, 18, 21, 23, 33, 41, 42, 46, 48, 49, 50, 55, 56, 59, 60, 72, 73, 74, 77, 78
variables, 15, 29, 119
vertical integration, 134
virology, 126
vision, 129, 135
vitamin A, 91

W

Washington, 9, 24, 62, 70, 79, 120
welfare, 127, 137
well-being, 127, 134
World Health Organization (WHO), 3, 7, 8, 9, 10, 24, 25, 34, 43, 44, 51, 52, 62, 68, 69, 70, 79, 93, 103, 104, 111, 120, 125, 126, 135
windows, 85, 113
workers, 52
World Bank, 9, 43, 52, 112, 120
worldwide, 7, 34, 42, 125, 135

Y

yellow fever, 126

Z

Zimbabwe, 3, 4, 8, 9, 10, 13, 14, 15, 22, 24, 25, 27, 28, 33, 35, 36, 40, 42, 43, 45, 46, 47, 49, 50, 51, 52, 55, 56, 62, 63, 64, 68, 69, 70, 71, 72, 77, 79, 83, 84, 92, 95, 96, 100, 101, 102, 103, 105, 106, 110, 111, 113, 114, 116, 117, 118, 119, 120, 125, 126, 129, 130, 131, 132